THE WAR ON MEDICAL TERRORISM

Why Single-Payer Medicare-for-All Is the
Cure for the U.S. Healthcare System

Les Stettner

iUniverse, Inc.
New York Bloomington

THE WAR ON MEDICAL TERRORISM

WHY SINGLE-PAYER MEDICARE-FOR-ALL IS
THE CURE FOR THE U.S. HEALTHCARE SYSTEM

iUniverse books may be ordered through booksellers or by contacting:

iUniverse
1663 Liberty Drive
Bloomington, IN 47403
www. iuniverse. com
1-800-Authors (1-800-288-4677)

ISBN: 978-1-4401-5808-7 (sc)
ISBN: 978-1-4401-5809-4 (ebook)
ISBN: 978-1-4401-5810-0 (hc)

Printed in the United States of America

iUniverse rev. date: 9/2/2009

Contents

Disregard Evidence-Based Medicine Because Practice Does Not Mean Perfect.

Do Not Pave the Way for Americans to Change Their Lifestyle.

Do Not Educate Americans on Alternative Care Options.

America Does Not Support Human Rights.

Socialize the Entire U. S. Healthcare System.

Ration All Healthcare-Related Services and Needs.

Take Away Our Freedom … Just Choose A, B, or Keep It the Way It Is.

Profile Everybody Living in America with Electronic Medical Records.

Do Not Change the Provider Reimbursement System.

Lobbyists and Private Interest Groups Should Decide Our Future.

Profit Must Drive All Medical Decisions.

You Have No Right to Healthcare or Any Rights at All.

Do Not Attempt to Take Ownership of Your Health.

Consumer Advocate for What?

Patient or Impatience? Supply and Demand Don't Matter.

Think Inside the Box with Catatonia, Not Dementia.

Do Not Invest in Your Health. Your Legacy Lives On.

How Much Time Do We Have Before We Are on Medicare?

Give Up and Be Defeated By Greed and Power.

About the Author

Les Stettner is an employee-benefits expert and the CEO of Longevity Benefits, an employee-benefits consulting company. Les is one of the country's leading authorities on health insurance. Les and his wife Danielle have two wonderful young children, Hailey and Dylan, and live in Parkland, Florida. Les is a former vice president of Aetna and Horizon Blue Cross and Blue Shield of New Jersey. Founded in 1999, Longevity Benefits is dedicated to helping its clients get the most out of our fragmented and uncoordinated healthcare system.

As an industry veteran, Les became frustrated by Congressional inactivity on reform and chose to channel his years of managed care experience into a viable solution to the American healthcare crisis. The goal of this book is to have the key creators of legislation read and absorb the suggestions of the book and to educate the American public on how to help themselves navigate the U. S. healthcare system. Les has the passion and experience to help improve the U. S. medical delivery system for all Americans. His unbiased approach, which emphasizes that an ounce of prevention equals a pound of cure, will surely help America cure its healthcare plague.

This book is dedicated to his mom, may she rest in peace, his dad, his wonderful loving family, and to world peace. Good health for all good people. We can do this together—united as one, sharing resources, and winning the war on sickness and disease. Les Stettner's next book is titled *One Plan: America's New Healthcare System.*

Mr. Stettner is a veteran of the health insurance field. Les has been licensed to sell life and health insurance since 1983. Mr. Stettner served as an officer for both Aetna and Horizon Blue Cross and Blue Shield of New Jersey. Writing this book is very self-sacrificial for Les since he is biting the hand that feeds him. In other words, Les has earned his living from health insurance commissions and from health insurance consulting for the past twenty-five years.

"The War on Medical Terrorism" is a call to action. The U. S. response to the flu scare from Mexico shows how fragmented our system is. We were still okay in a quasi-panic state, but it was scary. Quarantines or other containment issues are quite substantial—so are vaccines and medicine. The author wrote this book because his conscience could no longer get in the way of doing the right thing. If you are aging, sick, injured, aborted, or born in this country, you will experience the U. S. healthcare system.

Under the right healthcare system, all Americans will be aware of their genetic propensities and live healthy lives by remaining conscious of their healthcare and monitoring it. The best way to address sickness is to prevent it or know how your particular illness has been treated and which treatment recommendations resulted in the most successful outcomes. Many of your unpleasant experiences with our healthcare system will happen after the fact. Confusing billing and understanding your coverage will have you challenged for months—if not years. If you do not become a statistic and actually experience a favorable outcome, then you have experienced what is so great about the U. S. healthcare system.

Maybe the procedure should have employed some evidence-based medicine to stack the odds of the desired outcome in your favor, but in our procedure incentivized, crisis-oriented, fragmented medical system, we have come to expect this type of medical practice. There is complete autonomy with no or little accountability. Les only wishes the best health and a speedy recovery for anyone seeking medical services. If so, you may feel our medical system is without fault or unbelievably capable … and it *is* extremely capable. Unfortunately, the quality of our healthcare system is eroding—largely due to reimbursement methodology for medical services, poor plan designs, and administrative greed by health insurance companies. They have enjoyed a monopoly for years.

One cannot escape the need for health insurance in America. The odds of a successful outcome for most procedures performed in the United States are favorable. However, health insurance companies—through poor plan designs and controlling reimbursement to providers of care with only profit in mind—can keep you from getting the care you need. Americans have managed to grapple with their healthcare system's problems for decades.

Instead of progress, our healthcare system is in a state of regression. Runaway out-of-pocket costs are crippling those who access medical services. Medical advances are growing and innovation is fantastic, but they are not helping us in the most economical ways.

An internist recommended that Les use a statin drug due to age and family history. Instead of an extensive physical due to genetics, family history, age, and medical history—or perhaps because Les appears slender and is athletic—his now ex-internist felt compelled only to recommend prescribing a statin. Without knowing any better, Les concurred. Les is not a doctor.

Unfortunately, two months later, Les had two heart attacks that might have been avoidable. In fact, most heart attacks can be avoided. Do you know how much money that would save? Instead of a $5,000 physical—and that is a pretty extensive and expensive annual physical—Les had a $200,000 heart procedure. Do the math and apply that to the population of the United States with a propensity toward coronary heart disease.

Coronary artery disease is the leading cause of death in America—more so than cancer—but it is one of the most common illnesses to treat. Prevention could have saved Les the hassle, money, and struggle for his life. Our medical system is laden with so many perverse incentives because of how insurance companies reimburse for medical services. Les is alive because of the good in our medical system. The U.S. healthcare system is broken, but is still capable of amazing things. Even with Les's background, he felt lucky to have access to the care he received—even if it was expensive and wasteful.

To learn the true nature of the U. S. healthcare crisis, imagine Les leading you to a fix for the average working person or a single mom who has two young children and needs affordable healthcare. Les shows us why we are where we are and explains conceptually how to get where we need to be on healthcare reform. There are so many moving pieces, but Les brings it all back together. If the infrastructure of our tortured medical system fails, it could lead to uncontrollable fatalities. Healthcare must become an immediate priority in America.

We are losing our grip. Restructuring the medical reimbursement incentives around preventive care and a healthy lifestyle are essential to the sustained economic revival of the United States—now *and* in the future. Recognizing genetic propensities at birth could create more responsibility.

People used to fish for their dinners. Now, fish is the most expensive food because it has been deemed healthy. Where is our sense of social consciousness? If you want to help farmers, finance fish farms so we can all benefit from the expenditure. It is not a question of how many procedures we perform or endure, but how many procedures could be avoided due to the right incentives in the medical reimbursement methodology. Spending money is spending money. Whether it is on sale or not, a purchase is a purchase. Saving money is not consuming. Leading a healthier lifestyle is not consuming the miracle of the human body. A single-payer reimbursement system and one plan for all medical care will be a winner for all American citizens—not only utilizers or our wonderfully talented providers of care.

We could solve the illegal immigration problem by implementing one health plan for *every* American citizen. Is that too simple? The only losers are the greedy executives who only create wealth for themselves at a cost to your health and economic well-being and the illegal aliens who will be forced to apply for U. S. citizenship the way it is done in most sophisticated countries across the globe in order to access our medical system. You don't have to be employed by those executives to be affected by their greed disease.

Health insurance companies are stealing your provider's compensation and making medical care and pharmaceuticals more expensive for all Americans. Dirty rat bastards should rot in hell.

Remember what President Obama said when campaigning … healthcare should be a right. Les could not agree more. Let him show you how. Don't worry—he has not left out Big Pharma. Why don't they use their marketing budgets to lower the costs of prescriptions for all Americans? Social consciousness and morals can mix well with profit when it is fair for everyone.

Introduction

Should America continue the mistake of punishing those Americans in need while rewarding Americans in power—at the expense of her people's future? We are in very precarious times.

I am counting on President Obama to reverse many of the prior administration's fatal economic blunders. Ignoring the healthcare crisis in America will result in the next major bankruptcy if Congress and the president do not do something during this administration. Congress needs to ignore party lines and help the future of Americans for a change. Live the differences—but get the job done. Do it right and do not rush it. We can't afford more mistakes.

Health insurance is cheap in America. That doesn't make it a right. It can be much less expensive. It gets a lot more expensive if you don't have a job or get sick.

Do not attempt to scare me healthy ... my mortgage is cheaper and I am in default. Are you in default of your health through your lifestyle?

Is this a crisis or an opportunity? President Obama will make even more history by solving the biggest social problem affecting our economy.

Privatize or socialize? Where does the money come from? Are taxpayers going to bear the brunt of socialized medicine? Does every taxpaying citizen deserve an unfair shake? Why are taxpayers paying for the uninsured illegal immigrants? If Medicaid decreases its financial criteria to catch the folks in a financial squeeze, we should be able to insure the majority of our citizens. (Universal should only apply to U.S. citizens, right?) Should it be illegal not to carry health insurance?

Why don't you get it? It's by design? Do you have any responsibility in this? If you are healthy, why would you need this now? What about the state versus the feds? Consumer driven healthcare marks the end of an era—not the beginning of anything truly useful. If you know how to direct your own care, why do we need doctors? HMOs, PPOs, point-of-service plans, indemnity plans, and even supplemental plans can be used in many effective ways together, but they are not. Most people covered by health insurance don't even understand the plan design that they selected—or that has been selected *for* them in the case of group health insurance. They don't understand what an uncovered benefit is or what contribution levels are. They don't know if they should contribute before or after taxes. COBRA rights and continuation of coverage options should be clear to people who are forced to end their health insurance plan.

The quality of healthcare is not being addressed well by any health insurance company because they control reimbursement. That is a conflict of interest. Shouldn't the quality of care be measured by a third party and outcomes reported to all providers in their profession? That would provide information to enable providers to practice evidence-based medicine? Whose grave are the health insurance companies digging anyway? The high utilizers of their benefit plans have many options that have not been taught to them. It is important in the new era of health insurance or whatever protection we arrive at, that members are educated and learn how to use their plans effectively. Members will be citizens of America, right?

Can we live with a crisis-oriented medical delivery system? Can we still afford it? Is it taking over our economy? Not yet. How can we fix our current healthcare system to maintain its dignity and integrity as the most sophisticated medical delivery system of healthcare in the world? What is a consumer's part in changing our medical system for the good of all America?

Opportunities in Healthcare

- Technology can complement the flow of information.
- Information leads to education.
- Patients and doctors will benefit together using the flow of information.
- Many diseases can be completely avoided thru lifestyle changes.
- Medical advances are excellerating substantially.
- When you get sick, how do you know what medical services you need? What is medically necessary? Well, "I want it done" is what I say. After all, I am the consumer that is directing my care and you are paying for it. I don't feel that way because my premiums are as much as my mortgage. I am paying for it—or maybe I am uninsured? Transparency really uncovers a lot, doesn't it? Transparency shows us the reimbursement rate

for medical services. Sometimes you get what you pay for. How will an illness affect your family's financial future, your loved ones or your work productivity?

Can I afford to be sick? What is my employer doing to help me? What kind of protection do we have now? How will the system save me if I can't afford it any longer? Can I get health insurance protection when I am sick and unemployed—or is it too late? Thanks for no protection.

What can we do now to make the U. S. healthcare system better? It is a question worth asking and answering.

Take some personal responsibility.

- Exercise and diet appropriately. Nutrition is so important.

- Make your healthcare a priority. You are what you eat. Your health is your wealth. Why have these expressions survived the test of time?

- How can technology benefit us? Shouldn't all doctors who practice medicine be online with all health insurance companies that they do business with or all of the vendors in healthcare? Shouldn't all medical records be available online with a personal password so that when we access urgent or emergency care, the providers who are saving us are able to access critical information instantly? Shouldn't any doctor or provider of medical services be forced to carry malpractice insurance? It seems ancient and perverse to ask these questions of undeniably the most inefficient and expensive healthcare system in the world.

Public programs need help to eliminate fraud and its nasty attachments. Is the government really good at this? Are our social programs like Medicare, Medicaid and Healthy kids really good? Did you know that the U. S. government reimburses physicians and hospitals at a higher rate than health insurance companies do in America for employees who are offered group coverage or individual coverage, but provide this protection at fraction of the administrative charges applied by health insurance companies? Where is that extra money going? What message are we giving providers? The watchdog is sleeping and the greedy are getting richer at our expense. Does this sound familiar?

So what are you doing? What is your part? What is your responsibility? Why don't you care?

President Obama said that healthcare should be a right. I hope that I can help him accomplish that—and I make my living selling health insurance to corporations. Is it truly a right to live an unhealthy lifestyle that leads to being unhealthy, less productive, and more costly for those who participate in paying premiums for health insurance of any kind?

Should there be a penalty for those who inflict unhealthy lifestyle choices upon themselves that lead to disease? What about companies? What if it is psychological? Insurance doesn't reimburse for that. What about those truly in need? What about those American citizens who are born with birth defects, mental illness, diabetes, or other critical illnesses? Where is our social responsibility? Is it in oil or war? What about American rights in America?

Does your health insurance company's disease-management program help lower costs? What about a society embracing the concept of evidence-based medicine? How good is evidence-based medicine? The proof is in the pudding.

If it's my responsibility as a patient or member of the health plan who is accessing their benefits to know my plan and to use it effectively, why would I not be doing research to increase the probability of a successful outcome for my particular procedure or interaction with the medical system? Perhaps I don't have access to that information.

Why is a cup of coffee for five dollars more important than your health?

Part of the problem we are having is the concept of consumer-driven healthcare. Many doctors are giving up. We need them. *Consumers go to doctors because they do not know how to direct their care.* Selling consumer-driven care to the government and providers is foundationally irrational. It is all about health insurance industry marketing. Transparency that exposes cost is simply based upon supply and demand and not quality. I know because I consult to providers on their reimbursement contracts with health insurance companies. Once again, size matters. Quality is an afterthought. Control is in the wrong hands.

HEDIS (Health Education Data Information Set) is not enough and consumers do not understand the process. If you work for a health insurer, you might have a vague understanding. These are standards that are enforced by regulators on managed care aka health insurance companies and their providers that barely results in better outcomes—and less expensive care—because these standards do not make for better outcomes. They increase cost. The stamp of approval is like the road to hell being paved with good intentions. In the span of life, the supply-and-demand curve within healthcare and the American lifestyle are some of the most challenging issues.

America is the world's leader in medical advances. We have the best access to the most sophisticated healthcare anywhere in the world and—better yet—some of the best-trained practitioners in the world. Why is the system so messed up? This book explains how you can be part of the solution. I am convinced that President Obama and Congress must pass sweeping healthcare reform now. Healthcare reform should transform America into asingle-payer system, which will become the most important social legislation passed since LBJ and Congress passed the Social Security Act and created Medicare.

How to Use This Book

The purpose of this book is to wage war on the health insurance industry. Costs are out of control, and insurance plan designs are shifting the burden of our crisis-oriented, fragmented, and uncoordinated medical system on all Americans for profit. Where was their responsibility? Private managed care and consumer-driven models of care are about insurance and profit—*not* better medicine that produces better outcomes.

Managed care was about controlling utilization and reimbursement. It was never about managing care in the best interests of the patient. Insurance companies are not the doctors who treat us. Physicians are getting ripped off financially by the same folks who are stealing from us as consumers. The Centers for Medicare and Medicaid in Washington have administrative costs hovering around 4 percent. This is either fantastic or unbelievable.

If single-payer Medicare-for-all is the model for the new healthcare system, we ought to expect around an 8 percent operating budget, which is phenomenal. There will be no $50 million bonuses paid to health insurance CEOs or out or work executives that are forced to go to work for Uncle Sam. Expect costs to grow and be manageable when the government begins a Medicare-for-all system. Every American—including providers of care to patients—will win. Doctors will enjoy better reimbursements and healthcare will be less expensive. Everyone comes out a winner.

No other country with a similar size and population has ever had a medical system as amazing as ours. What is amazing about the U. S. healthcare system is access. Single-payer will lead to better care and better outcomes. A first, it will be harder for physicians to conform and extremely troubling for the health insurance industry, but the good will outweigh the bad. We have a plethora of options for care at our disposal—almost anywhere in our country. No other country has that. When we switch over to single-payer, we will realize efficiencies that will produce better outcomes at substantially lower costs. Doctors will make more money per procedure, Americans will be healthier, and costs will be much lower. Our way of life is being threatened by inside terrorists and—instead of adjusting so we can get stronger—we just keep doing the same old thing and getting manipulated. A single-payer model of American healthcare will set our spirits free. Let it be.

Chapter 1:
Regulate Rhymes with …
Execute?

America cannot hold off the overwhelming demand for healthcare. A healthcare-related terrorism attack would cripple our current healthcare and financial systems. The American healthcare system is easy prey; it's fragmented and badly broken. We are already being terrorized by inefficiency and medical errors. Do you know how many deaths occur each year as a result of medical errors?

Based on a recent report on medical mistakes from the National Academy of Sciences' Institute of Medicine, in its report, To Err Is Human: Building a Safer Health System, the IOM estimates that *44,000–98,000 Americans die each year not from the medical conditions they checked in with, but from preventable medical errors.* And you thought that 9/11 was serious. This happens each year to Americans.

If those statistics came from a terrorist attack, you would know. We are already being terrorized by ourselves, and the potential for additional fatal attacks from numerous outside sources is growing.

Are we junkies addicted to medical co-pays with no reality check? How can we stop this unbearable catastrophe waiting to happen? Can we have our cake *and* eat it? We need to work at staying healthy.

We are not junkies, but Americans are in need of some relief. Where is it going to come from? A $1 bacon cheeseburger with ketchup and mayo? I doubt it. If we spent half of the TARP money on our healthcare system, things might improve. However, before we start throwing more money at this problem, we need to make the right decisions on what our healthcare system really needs.

Attacks on the U. S. healthcare system are coming from everywhere. We thought we were armed, but it turns out we are just dangerous—to ourselves mostly and everybody else we touch. Thank goodness that many more Americans die from medical error than terrorist attacks on our soil. That does not make these statistics feel any better, does it?

The supply side is getting much smaller. Attention is required to address this, but to the rest of us, it means no medicine and fewer care providers. We need doctors who are trained in preventive and alternative care to practice medicine and get paid for it. Our best doctors need some recognition. We need to take an interest in our own health.

Americans need healthcare planning for life. Western doctors will be armed with tons of new electronic information, but they need to be trained in alternative medicine and to become better at diagnosing patients. Medicine may be an inexact science, but we have an unprecedented amount of useful information at our disposal that should result in much better outcomes.

America is on the verge of a catastrophic physician shortage.

American politics could help advance the Electronic Age and empower the Health Information Age to enable Americans to seek healthier lifestyle choices and improve treatment outcomes from our providers.

Healthier lifestyle choices will save the most money. The best ways are through education and prevention. What is in your healthcare future and how can you live it up and enjoy your freedom without getting sick?

Care providers are sick of getting ripped off. What is in it for them? No risk translates to no reward financially. Doctors and Americans fear changes that scare the heck of out them financially. However, I will show you how we can become healthier and how U. S. healthcare can improve, be less expensive, and produce much better outcomes. We need everyone on the same page. *All American citizens who consume medical care and all providers need to participate in reform.*

An ounce of prevention is worth a pound of cure. Do you know why that expression has survived the test of time? It is the future. It applies to everything.

Hospitals are being built all over the United States without anyone to staff them. Are hospital-based doctors the ones you want? Why not? How would you know? If the correct incentives permeated our entire healthcare system, hospital-based doctors would not be overwhelmed with crisis-oriented, procedure-driven medicine. Someone has to educate Americans about why healthcare reform is stalled. This book might educate you and enable you to protect yourself. Self-defense is about protecting what you love—*not* being violent toward others. Adopt a healthier existence.

The costs of Band-Aids to the U. S. healthcare system have been devastating. Health insurance companies continue to behave irresponsibly toward insureds and the entire provider side of medicine. So do pharmaceutical companies. America's healthcare delivery system is sinking to new lows and we are afraid of evolving. Some horrible monster sociopath is thinking of America's demise and our healthcare system is our single biggest weakness. We are not prepared. We need some defense before we launch the offensive on our bodies.

Sound familiar? Haven't Americans procrastinated about the healthcare problem for years?

I am not bashing the U. S. healthcare system; we need to heal the system—or what's left of the most sophisticated healthcare delivery platform in the world. It still is and always will be. Now let's make it better than ever—so our entire population can benefit from a more humane approach to healthcare.

Our healthcare system has the potential to dwarf any other country's measured outcomes in healthcare-delivery statistics. What we need is leadership and an open mind. Yes, it will take money, leadership, and desire—but what better investment is there to make in America's future? Wall Street? What about life? Are capitalists cold? No, so straighten out before you ruin it for everybody here. American citizens need your help, Uncle Sam. Life is about living, making the right decisions, and planning for the future. Don't you need your health to realize your potential? We are among the most productive people in the world, but we're stressed out of our minds.

Doesn't a Cuban have a longer life expectancy than an American does?

I don't mean the cigar. It's too close considering the per capita costs of U. S. healthcare delivery. Americans deserve the right to have high expectations from our medical system. Americans once took pride in our medical system. Now all we have is gay pride. No insult is intended, as I except people for whom they are. Where is our dignity? Where is the cure for AIDS and many cancers? Most likely, the cure is right around the corner if not already available.

Every American citizen should have healthcare—not free healthcare—but the right to healthcare as suggested by President Obama prior to being elected. The opportunity is now or—as Hillary found out—never. Deadlocked, partisan politics will destroy America's future and the only people with jobs won't get the job done, again. That is why you need to be aware now.

Who is terrorizing the U. S. healthcare system? Where is all the money going?

Chapter 2:
How Can We Reduce the Cost of Healthcare In America? It's My Life and I Will Do What I Want To.

America can reduce healthcare costs by *50 percent* whenever we are ready—even with our current problems.

Why doesn't it happen? Come on, you can't be that naïve.

Have you ever asked yourself what would happen should you get really sick and need to use your healthcare plan? Will your claims even be paid? My non-English-speaking HMO doctor may give me an appointment and help me direct my care if I am insured—*if* they remember to treat me after I wait in their office for an hour. Am I possibly better off with my dog's compassionate veterinarian? They still speak English over there. Is English still America's native language? If you can read this book in English, then you ought to be able to communicate with your doctor in English. By the way, my dog's vet does not require concierge medicine to treat my dog—even though he is busy and has a great reputation. I wonder why?

My vet still gets a fee for services provided. Reimbursement incentives are all wrong in medicine. A risk model for providers designed to keep us well throughout our lives would help. Providers can be rewarded for keeping us well, but that just makes too much sense. What if you are already sick? It still works.

If you are like most Americans with health insurance, you are broke without a kiss, financially. Worried about paying your mortgage? Worry about your healthcare premiums. Premiums are outrageous, and there is so much cost-shifting in most health insurance plan designs that getting sick or being sick in America is very expensive to all. Out of pocket costs due to medical interaction are crippling Americans financially.

Medical-related bankruptcies are at an all-time high. Health insurance premiums are a huge strain on people's budgets. Corporations are going out of business due to poor economic policy and the costs of their benefit plans, as well as administration. We can help American businesses create jobs by addressing this beast called healthcare.

Medical reimbursement is smitten with perverse incentives. Medicare is full of fraud, yet it holds the key to advanced incentives for Universal Care. So do you as an American citizen.

Americans without health insurance—including business owners to non-taxpaying illegal immigrants and murderers in prison—may very well be better off than the average American sucker that has health insurance protection. Do you want to know why that is the case?

Because the uninsured population does not pay premiums and we do for the same services. Do you have something to lose? Can you pay? Do you know your current health profile? Do you care? Try another $1 bacon cheeseburger and fries. That will do wonders for your arteries. Why not do something to help yourself that doesn't cost money? Ever think about it?

Do you want confidentiality? Why? Who and what do you need protection from? Health insurance underwriting knows a completely different story when they are cherry picking health risks for their company to insure. In addition to cost, that is one of the major problems with individual coverage. Costs are low if you are perfectly healthy, but it all hits the fan when you get sick.

Imagine if they could look at your genetic profile to determine your risk … no one would ever qualify for insurance coverage. Underwriters and their insurance company have access to all of your confidential medical information. Guaranteed issue community rating is not a federal mandate though it should be. That would mean that any American who needed and could pay for health insurance would be guaranteed to qualify for it, and the premiums would be the same among all age groups. It is available in certain states in America, but health insurance was turned into a State phenomenon due to the McCarron-Ferguson Act almost fifty years ago. That is why plans are different in every state. The lack of standardization has resulted in extreme confusion. Under single payer, McCarron Ferguson would be repealed.

Guaranteed issue community rating would spread the risk and make health insurance available to all. It might cost a touch more than it is today, but it is already too late for that. Insurance companies say it costs too much because it costs *them* too much. There won't be enough money for that seven-figure multimillion-dollar bonus or the deplorable greed that permeates the top earners of the health insurance industry—let alone enough jobs.

Making money and being a capitalist is wonderful—as long as you add value to society, do not rip off your fellow citizens, and do the right thing for America. There is not enough money for huge, unjustified bonuses. We should do whatever the insurance company says to do to shore up their profit-making machines, reserves, or add to their general and administrative expenses. That has been the trend. You sign applications and contracts that allow risk takers to pry into your healthcare data to determine your personal health-risk profile. If you don't comply, the health insurance company will not cover you—or they will offer you protection with riders or preexisting conditions exclusions. So much for protection and guaranteed issue when insurance companies always say that community rating and guaranteed issue coverage will cost more. That is because health insurance companies are in control. They make policy in Washington. Health insurance companies own our politicians and their minds. Only when it serves their interests will you even know your health profile exists and is available to them. By the way, if you are sick and the risk takers, a. k. a. health insurance companies, offer you protection—watch out! The renewal premiums will reflect their cherry picking or they will get you next year in some other way such as changing how they cover pharmaceuticals. They usually just add huge premium increases to cover their manipulation in an attempt to make money.

President Obama never really had a health plan. He, McCain, and Kennedy never had a leg to stand on—let alone a healthcare reform platform. At least President Obama recognizes that healthcare should be a right. It's not an original idea, but it is the right answer. I hope his natural leadership abilities can circumvent the usual Congressional obstacles and execute this fundamental change without all of us getting ripped off in the process. President Obama's party currently controls Congress. The road to healthcare reform has been paved for President Obama. We can be thankful that the new Health and Human Services Secretary may have more of an open mind and can accomplish what the president wants to see happen. Obama has to make a careful choice— one that makes sense. I believe that he has. A bipartisan approach will work when the result is better outcomes all the way around. Job growth, more efficiency, and better results would be helpful. Politics are so divisive, too. We need to bring it all back together. We are in a crisis. That is when Americans are like no other country. Americans have an uncanny ability to come together in a crisis like no other people in the world. We will resolve this healthcare crisis.

You should know that anything can happen to your health— regardless of your age, lifestyle, or genetics. The idea is to stack the odds in your favor instead of someone else's. There are companies that can give you your personal genetic profile for only $399. It is amazing how far technology is taking us. That genetic profile report may provide the impetus to strive for lifestyle changes while being raised by your parents because they will know what can contribute to your health and vitality and opposed to the things that will hurt you.

Lifestyle, genetics, and prevention will fuel the changes that will develop healthcare delivery at its potential here in America.

They say that 98 percent of all heart attacks can be prevented. I don't know about you, but I would rather prevent one than end up sick in a hospital with a heart attack. It may not happen that way, but we can try. I have a great idea for prevention. Start by taking an interest in your health. There is more to do.

Can you believe in this day and age that health insurance is not guaranteed issue everywhere in the United States? The concept is barbarian. Health insurance companies have been getting away with murder and stealing from providers and consumers since the managed care movement and model of healthcare delivery. Confidentiality is almost impossible—so let's work on punishing those who use other people's confidential information against them. It is discrimination. So are medical underwriting and pre-existing conditions clauses in health insurance contracts. Without these protections, the health insurance companies will no longer be able to carry absurd operating costs and pay multimillion-dollar bonuses. Either way, we need to do away with medical underwriting in order to get a truly universal fix for medical coverage.

Does it really matter? Yes. When an underwriter is denying you coverage because of a pre-existing condition, the underwriter is doing their job. Size matters to them. If you are big and fat, you are statistically undesirable. What kind of equality is that? Do you mean that physical size—with which one monopolizes a room with—is not to their advantage?

What kind of rhyme or reason is there in penalizing the sick and unhealthy?

The United States fights for every other country's human rights and freedom. Let's hear it for Americans for a change. Americans need Uncle Sam to do the right thing for a change. That is change. What is not change is a very familiar-looking cast of characters who managed to set the precedent for how to unravel the world's economies. President Obama spoke about change, so let's do it. Why can't we reach out and help our own citizens? America needs jobs and taxes for healthcare reform. Healthcare is not free.

What rights are we fighting for right here at home in America?

Confidentiality is BS in the Wild West of the Internet!

Do you have something to hide? I doubt it. Are you purposely hurting anyone? Can any hacker find out everything about you? The answer is probably yes. So move on. If you are breaking the law, someone will find out eventually.

Since when has there not been a consequence for every action? That applies to eating, smoking, not exercising, and other bad things for your health.

Does confidentiality really matter? It matters to unlawful people who are willing to take that chance.

When it comes to discrimination, confidentiality makes a big difference. "I don't want any fat, unhealthy, drug-infested losers working for me." But, if they are the best person for the job, Mr. Executive, you probably should hire them. Otherwise without proof against them, that attitude borders on discrimination!

Small-minded CEOs do not create jobs; they lose them but come out financial winners at the cost of the common man. That seems to be a pattern among today's CEOs. Track records are not reflected in company stock prices.

Entrepreneurs create opportunity; monopolies often destroy opportunity.

Monopolies are greedy, and the majority of them are laying off thousands of workers to shore up their financial books. This is great for balance sheets—but not good for short-term job growth.

What kind of leadership is that? Not the kind that can overcome the global competitiveness that we created. Sometimes you get what you wish for.

Be prepared for the upcoming battle on healthcare. Too many powerful stakeholders are lobbying to keep you from learning the truth. They have surrounded Washington with their powerful lobbies and have more access to President Obama than any of us do.

It is disappointing to see what is going on in Washington, but I am hopeful that President Obama cleans it up for the good of all Americans. Know who the players are and what the stakes are. Think change. Think socialized medicine—just kidding.

Single-payer is about diverting the money we pay for health insurance premiums in to healthcare itself. Stop worrying about what healthcare reform is called. "Single Payer" is simply a method of reimbursement. There is so much more to do.

Would you rather continue to see costs spiral upward and CEOs financially rape consumers and doctors. What do you choose? I choose healthcare itself, which can be accomplished through a single-payer, Medicare-for-all model. Let me show you how.

Think preventive care, exercise, eating healthily, and making an effort to stay or get healthy. You have to think green to be lean. You must have a personal commitment to your health in order for America to be successful in the War on Medical Terrorism. We all bleed red and basically want the same things. Americans all want to be healthy and financially stable in this wonderful land of opportunity.

Did you notice that the 2008 presidential candidates stopped talking about innovative healthcare solutions and how they would get there? Ah … maybe because they had no idea? Reform without details is not reform. Finally, President Obama is making the subject a priority. Is it all about money? No way, mind you that the politicians tend to tell you we can't afford it. That is right. We can't afford to keep it the way it is. We can make it with a prayer. Middle-class Americans are taking it on the chin. Do something, please. Stimulate what we need—more jobs with futures and staying healthy—not financial arrangements to shore up balance sheets so that it is business as usual. Address this financial crisis to avoid the next one.

Psssssssst … This is confidential info …

Chapter 3:
What Could Make Healthcare Better in America? If You Don't Know Where You Are Going, Any Road Will Take You There.

If you are a team player, you will benefit from this book. It is about empowerment, evolution, and effect.

What a farce American efforts in human rights around the globe appear to be when we can't even benefit from a humane healthcare system that treats all of our American citizens equally and with reasonable affordable choices.

American "seniors" and "the poor" may take Medicare and Medicaid for granted, but they sure as hell are glad that they have it when they need it. Sometimes the medical system itself fails in these two social healthcare programs—not the degree of protection that these programs yield to Americans in need. The VA has served an excellent purpose. Many complain that it is not up to date. What an abomination since those veterans that use it fought for our freedom—which is something that most Americans take for granted.

Healthcare for terminally ill elderly Americans is inhumane. Did you know that 27 percent of Medicare expenditures are spent on end-of-life care? Forget the quality of life from a healthcare standpoint. If U. S. healthcare can keep you alive—whatever your quality of life—we endorse it. It is unrealistic and unfair to the most vulnerable.

Euthanasia must be a choice for the terminally ill. When you have no choice, the medical system and its providers get to torture you. That is not good medicine—it's just expensive and unaffordable medicine.

There are several arguments against abortion and euthanasia. The pro-choice model is the only one that makes modern-day sense. If you believe in God, then you probably feel that God created all medicine —good *and* bad. The two subjects are largely not related, but removing pain and suffering in some cases explains some of the opinions. Nobody with a brain would ever promote abortion as a method of birth control, and no decent person would ever promote death to a healthy person. It is not right for social injustices to promote religion or other illogical reasoning to take away choice.

What good is suffering? Some would say that grieving relatives or loved ones or doctors and hospitals benefit from keeping you alive at any expense—regardless of the quality of your life. I guess it is a way to make a living. Healthcare is a personal responsibility that we need to do the most with. America needs to be fair to the elderly and provide them with choice—not healthcare at any expense as the only choice. All protection has its limitations. The government and a health insurance company already offer limited plan provisions. Yes, your health plan does not cover everything you would like it to and there is some cost sharing. Uncle Sam is not going to decide who gets care and who does not. Logic and maturity need to apply to advanced medical procedures that cost outrageous amounts of money. We can do better. More effective standards of care can be established.

Medicare needs to be updated financially to reflect medical innovation, but its longevity as a social welfare program to seniors—who learned to become dependent upon the system by design—has been astonishing and must be preserved. Thank you, President Johnson. Medicare has been a remarkable achievement—considering the despicable attempts by private enterprise and free markets that have succeeded at ripping off the government, hence American citizens. We need it and want it. Retirement with financial security is part of the American dream. Those of us that pay our share and dues expect it. Medicare contributions from income are an investment in our social security.

Congress could build on the Medicare model and grant the right of healthcare to all Americans—but that would be too easy. Creating a Medicare-for-All model that emphasizes prevention and is followed through with providers at risk makes sense. The cream will rise to the top and the reimbursement and practice incentives will change. That is how we can empower the best doctors to help Americans reach our healthcare potential.

What we need here in America is another financial crisis—this time from the health insurance sector. How about more billionaires as a result of it, rewarding useless peter-principled executives by creating sicker, poorer Americans that they will choose to ignore? What about a terrorist attack at a biological level? Are we ready? No way. Fragmentation will spread the risk of disease. We are not doing our homework. How do we prepare?

A bailout is not socialism; it is communism. Pitiful! It is all a conspiracy against the vulnerable, our children. What happened to capitalism and survival of the fittest? Everyone is out for themselves. What happened to being a team player? There are too many fast food dollar menus. Do you even know the difference between what is healthy to eat and what is not? There is so much wonderful information at our fingertips on the Internet. Drinking soda instead of water will rot your teeth and make you gain weight. Anything in moderation won't kill you. What about the benefits of living healthily? Why worry if you think the world is coming to an end? It is not ... so wake up and start feeling good.

What value are these health insurance companies CEOs bringing to the table? Short-lived profits at an unbearable cost to middle-class working Americans who are striving to live the American dream under the direction of some greedy evil genius CEO? Is that who is creating—I mean losing—jobs in America? Just look at where the jobs are disappearing in the health insurance industry and what kind of service these organizations now provide. The future of health insurance in America looks bad. Look at the overall five-year compensation of the top healthcare executives. Where is their moral fiber not to mention the supposed protection they market that is more fraudulent than protective in many cases?

E-mail me; I have so many examples that I could write another book on just the horror cases I have seen. They happen everywhere—yes, even in America. (lsx100@yahoo. com)

Many Americans have endured over and over again and still became castaways in the land of opportunity. Bad health steals their chances. If you are healthy, chances are you don't know how lucky you are and will take it for granted. Live long, prosper, and have a healthy life. Be happy and bring out the best in yourself and others.

What will the health insurance filibusters and lobbyists do to make a living—or Congressman for that matter—if we fix everything? Do you think they should get a real job? How about making America as good as it could be? That is why we elect and hire them, isn't it?

Who would there be to influence or manipulate you in some clever way? Leave it to the health insurance companies and their bought-off bureaucrat friends. They will find a way. Are we doomed?

Now you understand why health insurance companies are stealing your money. They are terrorists. Whether you are a doctor or a consumer you need to know.

Who can you trust more?

Dysfunctional public servants doing a supposed thankless job to protect Americans … lucky knuckleheads with no accountability and a Democratic Congress or some cutthroat, evil, greedy, genius freaks, who know how to squeeze every dollar out of our fragmented healthcare system into profit? The average health insurance company CEO and their respective companies pocket 25 percent to as much as 50 percent of every healthcare dollar from those in need of care. They are leaving our freedom vulnerable. The best defense is prevention.

Why isn't anybody talking about the new American healthcare system? I have a new health plan. I cannot share it with you in this book, but I will tell you that my health plan is universal and prevention-focused. It will not cost more, but it will create positive change that will help put American industry back to the forefront of innovation—where they should be. Congress is talking around healthcare. Healthcare expenses are barely understood, yet the U. S. economy is extremely tied into healthcare. U. S. healthcare protection will all come down to:

Insurance companies or the government?

Free and overregulated markets or single-payer medicine in the United States?

Perception is reality. Whether or not you like everything the way it is won't matter. President Obama will be in for the fight of his life. I hope he is up for it. Nothing in the healthcare world is standing still. The wrong people are advising the president on healthcare. Most of the advice is coming from CEOs that are not adding value to the system—just to their pockets. We will become victims financially and at a huge cost to American health if that is where the advice comes from.

With any luck, President Obama will lay the groundwork for change prior to implementing major reform. This change needs to be everlasting.

Would it be easier to understand one plan design for all Americans instead of the thousands of plan designs that exist today? You bet it would. Imagine completely understanding your healthcare benefits. One plan ... Medicare-for-All.

Forget the scare tactics of Canadian or European socialized medicine in the United States because much of it is untrue and would never exist here. Access to care is better in the United States than any other country and can stay that way under single-payer. Free markets and capitalism will complement single-payer through innovation in the new U. S. healthcare system. That is the beauty of it. Lost jobs will be replaced with jobs that have a future and are serving and contributing to the best long-term interests of the USA.

The United States cannot be compared to any other country for the purposes of transitioning the only medical system in the world like it to a more effective, efficient model of healthcare, which should not be a take away from Americans. In the United States, there is easy access to many of the best medical institutions in the world from almost any populated area. You can get an MRI or other tests usually within miles of any suburban location. Access doesn't stop Americans from accessing the care they need; it is their insurance company, their health, or lack of money.

Although our tax money is rebuilding transportation systems in other countries while ours falls apart, we can still get around pretty easily. President Obama is addressing some of these issues in the stimulus package. If you are scared of anything, you should be frightened of the fact that doctors and medical services are going to be hard pressed to accommodate upcoming demand from baby boomers, their children, and their children's children.

Common sense fact: It is much less expensive to administrate one plan from one company instead of thousands of plans from hundreds of insurance companies.

The facts that support this are all over the place. Gosh. Maybe if the practice of medicine wasn't such a complicated hassle for doctors governed by your managed care company, there would not have been such a mass exodus of our most talented doctors, who help future doctors learn at our finest teaching hospitals.

Our medical system is in shambles and no one wants to admit it. The legal system is a small part of the problem. It is laden with its own issues. Good health must be part of the law. We need to mandate it.

Sweat the small stuff because it is your money being stolen by monopolies. Trickle-down economics is history. The deceit is in the details. I am a health insurance consultant, consumer advocate, and physician-contracting consultant. This is how I feed my family. I have been licensed in the healthcare field more than twenty years. In many ways, this book is self-sacrificial. I want to do the right thing. We need to help productivity in America. Most insurance brokers have very little experience in insurance policies and are useless. If you are picking an insurance broker, you should use the same care and judgment that you would to select an attorney.

Healthcare isn't only about the uninsured or the poor. Those numbers of 47 million uninsured Americans are deceiving. Ten million of those uninsured Americans are earning more than $50,000 per year. Ten million more of those qualify for Medicaid and are not seeking it. The U. S. government should be seeking them. Ten million more of those uninsured are illegal immigrants. Don't let all of the political lies that manipulate your perception keep you from realizing the truth. I deal with the insured people of this country, and they are dissatisfied with where healthcare costs and services are going.

The taxpaying citizens of the United States employ the government. They work for us. So, I ask you again … who can you trust … your own employees who are paid to represent your best interests all of the time or some company from the private sector that takes risk and is focused on profit before care and reimbursement? Sometimes answers and solutions are right in front of us.

I know that you can't believe how gullible you have been.

Companies may have boards of directors that oversee operations and can hire and fire chief executives, but they are more focused on profit than on you and your healthcare. Boards of directors of huge monopolies often threaten top executives with the "do a good job speech (get the stock price up) or else we will give you a $200 million exit bonus and you can become some other company's problem." Normally, that would be no big deal and we all get it. The private enterprises should be producing a profit or adding to reserves at a reasonable cost of doing business and running like a finely greased machine. Executive performance-based incentives are rarely based on generosity toward insureds. There is no direct correlation between what health insurance chief executives earn and how good a job they do. The stock price drives the quality of a company, right? These are not socially conscious folks. They are part of the axis. Sweeping legislation should come their way—and quickly.

Did you know that federal employees have the American public paying for their health coverage or a portion of it in the FEHBP or Federal Employees Health Benefits Program, which offers a plethora of alternatives for coverage from the nation's largest health insurance companies? It is still a big financial rip-off. Some protection is better than no protection.

What a privilege it is to work for Uncle Sam. I will probably end up being a Medicare fraud watchdog or in some other government position because I can save the great people of this country—including me—from being ripped off. What a pathetic showing. I have a plan that will work and provide the right incentives to providers and consumers. It is an investment in the future that will have a huge payoff to our country's citizens. It is our obligation to our children to leave them a better country—not a debt-laden sinking ship.

Even the FEHBP health insurance plans have their design flaws. They are getting more expensive to the employees through plan design changes that continue to cost shift an overwhelming financial burden to the unlucky heavy utilizers of the healthcare plan. Americans can get sick. We don't have to incentivize it or live that way. The nation's largest employer—the government—has a lot of influence in many ways that impacts how their employees' claims are treated by the respective participating insurance company. Insurance companies can't afford to lose the government as an account. Therefore, federal employees are better off than any of us that work for a small employer. Small employers are dropping health insurance at an alarming rate. Health insurers only allow the sale of association health insurance plans to monopolies like themselves—such as the AARP—that have similar political ambitions and to some large staffing companies.

When businesses try to band together legally as an association, the massive lobbying efforts of health insurance companies shut them down because it was cheaper than losing their most profitable block of business and control. It is too bad that the top ten major health insurers spend hundreds of millions to keep association plans from becoming another alternative. Small businesses can't afford their premiums unless they band together to be considered a large group in order to get some rate or premium relief. I understand why the insurance companies don't want association business. Based upon our current underwriting and actuarial assumptions, almost every multi-employer, non-homogenous group such as an illegal MEWA or an association will eventually turn sour from a claims standpoint. Most insurance companies have little or no association business on the books and continue to prevent their formation— regardless of their political positions. Small business loses again. Seniors don't even realize that they can buy a federally standardized supplemental insurance plan from many competitors of AARP and sometimes at a much lower premium. Seniors enroll in Medicare Advantage plans and don't even know what it is or who pays for what.

United Health Group is the underlying insurer to AARP's supplemental medical plans. AARP serves an excellent purpose. United Health is having difficulties getting their different organizations in sync and does not have its act together. I do a lot of business with them. Americans could be the victims of their demise should they be unsuccessful. The U. S. government may have to bail them out. That means you and me—akin to GM and Ford and Chrysler or the banks. If current trends continue, they will be one of the first major health insurance companies at the TARP window of disaster relief along with some of their competitors.

The U. S. Healthcare Crisis is coming. What can we do?

We are already in a crisis, but we're not in crisis mode. What really happens to your health insurance claims?

When an insurance company receives your claim, its software is designed to look for ways to pend the claim (delay the processing of it) or deny it completely. At the start of a policy, when an insurance company underwrites or examines risk, they always start with the glass half empty for the policyholder. The doctor or providers submit codes to determine their reimbursement. They deserve to be compensated for the services they provide. The idea is to make money from the risk-taking business—which is fine, but just not in healthcare. This is a fundamental issue that capitalism never dealt with. There were too many opportunities for abuse from those with power. Now look at the mess these Americans have created for other Americans.

Healthcare should be redesigned to take into account the current problems and where fixing them will take us.

The U. S. healthcare system could cut their costs in half almost immediately by making a few constructive changes on reform.

Insurance companies are profit-driven, capitalistically engaged entities, and they behave that way. The risk-takers have their extremely important part in all societies. They make money just holding on to premiums and making payees wait unjustifiably long for their reimbursement (the float). Why do you think the doctor or hospital makes you sign all of those forms regarding payment? Health insurance companies are like a bank that owns your money and takes a risk that is highly stacked in their favor ... sounds like Las Vegas or a Ponzi scheme.

Do you want to wager on your personal health? Is it too late?

- Americans are becoming deadbeat medical patients.
- We don't pay medical bills.

- We take un-prescribed medicines.

- We don't live healthy lifestyles.

- We can be physically and mentally out of control.

- We can be irresponsible.

- We can be immoral.

- When did you last see your dentist? Are you foreclosing on your health? Did you brush and floss your teeth thoroughly this morning because you have chronic halitosis? I know that dental hygiene doesn't come easy to you, but the plague in your mouth corrodes your heart, fatman.

You're smoking after being diagnosed with Chronic Onset Pulmonary Disease. Gee … Isn't that how you got it in the first place, chimney face? COPD … You just saw a commercial on TV for it. You can take a pill now. With any luck, your heart will give out first … or just maybe they can rebuild you. Get the pharmaceuticals off the air and put the marketing money into lowering the costs of pharmaceuticals. The doctors who prescribe medicine need to be targets of marketing—not the consumers.

My friend who just went in for a transplant said, "Ah, it feels so good. I can pollute my body again. I can live. It is like being born again."

A transplant is a sort of cleansing. It's not fun to be subject to the procedure—especially if it could have been prevented. That's the ticket to good health—like the stimulus bill will do for our economy. Transplant all of my core body parts that allow me to function both physically and mentally so I can lead the carefree lifestyle. Who needs care when we have the marvels of modern medicine to help us? Obviously this sick American is not a team player.

While you are paying the bill for my transplants, did anyone ever tell you that you are what you eat? The metamorphosis of the human genetics will surely mutate mankind because of some sickoid terrorist trying to get a partial prepayment from those seventy-two virgins they told him about. America is not ready. Why does everyone hate each other? We are all people. Religion is the root of this evil. We all start out as innocent babies to be partitioned by religion and color. Instead of faith, we develop hatred through prejudice. They can sew all of our stomachs smaller, lipo-suck our fat out, and rat poison our wrinkles away. They can reconstruct our body parts and why the hell not? Genetic reengineering, control, chaos, and whatever—it's a party on your dollar. Remember that what goes around comes around—when you least expect it. Genetic reengineering scares most people. However, what if it is for the good of mankind? Can we take what is broken and fix it? Can we regulate it? Are we safe?

Drugs, sex, and rock and roll—bring it on baby. Robin Hood or someone else can pay for it. Do you have to pay those vulgar medical bills that are in collections? You know the ones you thought you had insurance to pay for only to find out that you did not.

How sweet it is to indulge your sweet tooth—now that your sugar is raging and the holes in your teeth need filling. You can take a pill for diabetes or whatever, but teeth are already replaceable if you can afford it. Is it all about money? There is no doubt that money has something to do with it. Money is attached to higher education.

Fatty foods are in. Fat is in. Fat bellies stick out at the beach. Last week I saw a really pretty pregnant girl about twenty years old.

It turned out that she was just fat. There were hardly any fat girls in my high school. Today, high cholesterol and diabetes are in. Dollar menus and fast food are everywhere—in your body and mind that is. We can always get new body parts. I always thought those preservatives would keep us alive forever. Doesn't it seem like the drug companies are financing the fast food companies? Are you listening out there? Penalize them. They are killing us.

Indiscretion comes so easy to us—but at what cost? What else can we do to mess it all up. You are what you eat, porker.

Whatever happened to that deadbeat patient?

You are right here. It is so easy to find you—eating fatty foods and sitting on your fat butt while your body is getting sicker and sicker so you can impose your sick fat ass on our medical system for free and create medical debt. Yeah ... that is it. You must love medical debt. It is always nice to get something for nothing—especially when it comes to your health. What are we going to do—put you in jail? Okay ... that is a great deal. Free healthcare, room and board, cable TV ... all for not paying your medical expenses. I love this county. Can't we do better than that?

Why take care of yourself when someone else can do it for you for free? Educate Americans and penalize the killers. Let's start a good health holiday week in America called the "optimum health week" to use the words of the great author Andrew Weil.

You are so sick. You can't afford your medicine because your crack habit comes first. You can't even see the doctor because you can't afford the cab ride to get there. No one will give you a break. You owe your body some cures, but your ills are taking you over. You are dysfunctional. That sucks.

You know what to do, but you can't do anything about it. You are the deadbeat patient and have mental stumbling blocks that you cannot overcome without help. You can't help your body or your mind. You can't pay your bills, and you won't take your doctor's advice. You do nothing because you are so irresponsible. You are totally disabled from head to toe. You need to help yourself. We should be helping you too because you are burdensome instead of productive to society.

Just got out of surgery ... have to tell everybody that you ... couldn't wait to get out of there ... everyone was sick in there. You can't believe how many medical bills you have been tossing in the garbage. Collection agencies are chasing you down. You got the better of American generosity through Uncle Sam, and you don't appreciate it. We won't find you because you are the rambling man doing the best one can to be invisible and not pay the bill. Single-payer is the only thing that can stop you in your tracks. A new system of identification of citizenship that will grant you access to U. S. medical care should exist and be a possible solution to immigration issues. Address two issues at once?

No wonder your doctor is always complaining about the insurance companies to you.

The negative impact that insurance companies have had on the way medicine is practiced today is a direct reflection of the damage that insurance companies have caused. Managed care stopped short of its original idea, which was to control cost and improve quality. It was a very flawed model of health insurance plan design that has done much more damage than good. Consumer-driven care is much worse.

Consumer awareness and education about health is much better than knowing what a procedure you need costs and trying to pick the least expensive route or not do it at all. What a great model of care.

Medicine is not about the patient ... it is about the profit.

Our legal system has created a self-fulfilling incentive to argue every point in a health insurance contract subject to many varying interpretations. What a system. The more the legal system gets involved in healthcare and complicates it, the worse our medical system will perform on your behalf. In Florida, many doctors don't even carry malpractice insurance. Should they be allowed to practice without insurance? Not everything in America is perfect ... but it is damn good. That's probably why we have so many illegal immigrants. Plus, they don't pay for healthcare. They just get it through our emergency rooms. They don't pay taxes. They just send their hard-earned money back to their countries where they are from. They sacrifice to save money which seems foreign to many of us in America.

America—like every other country in the world—has lots of room for improvement. Only now, we have more competition. America did very well in the 2008 Olympics, didn't we? We are still America ... the greatest country in the world. Stand up for yourself.

When the government pays your medical claims, it looks for ways to pay timely regardless of profit. Our regulators actually have rules for how much time can elapse before a claim is paid. The private sector always proves the government is stupid until they catch up with them. The government overpays for Medicare and Medicaid claims to a number of suppliers, providers, and others who service the medical industry, which is a different problem completely. It is called fraud and lack of proper oversight. *It is not about more regulations—it is about the appropriate enforcement.* Seniors and most of the insureds are billed by providers—even though they are covered for the medical services they received. They are often double- and triple-billed and go into collections before time and aggravation is exhausted. After all, it is private industry that has been committing fraud on the government.

The U. S. government commits fraud on its employer—the American people. The payer is the loser, most of the time. When fraud is committed by the private sector against the government with regard to public programs like Medicare and Medicaid, the damage is shared among all citizens through wasted tax money. That is where some of your grocery money is going. Besides, it is a white-collar crime that can be avoided through improved and more authoritative federal oversight. I wish I could afford to volunteer to clean it up.

Taxpayers do not have to get ripped off on healthcare when we fix the system. There is so much to be gained for every American—rich or poor. Good health is a privilege and does not only belong to the rich.

It is nice to know that the 2008 presidential candidates both agreed that if their insurance is good enough for Congress then it should be good enough for you, too.

So we may be getting something as opposed to nothing if Congress ever chooses to seriously debate healthcare reform again. Because the economy is on very shaky ground, it becomes the next diversion or dog-waggin' road to nowhere. In other words, little progress will be accomplished by Congress thru rushed legislation which doesn't address the most critical aspects of reform.

The political agenda talks the rhetoric of reform. There was little reform in either candidate's proposal. More broken Band-Aids will not work. Where are the facts?

Two rich, lucky, educated men that ran for president think that access to overpriced insurance protection is the answer to the problems that plague our healthcare system. Don't we ever learn from our mistakes?

How ignorant can we be to ignore this issue? Just listen to our politicians. Finger-pointers are not leaders unless they resolve issues. I have some solutions that I will unveil in this book. No one has a monopoly on the right answer.

The government might not always represent your current thinking, but make no mistake about it, our congressmen and the president of the United States work for the citizens of our country.

They may hurt us from time to time with bad decision making, but their hearts are always in the right place. Even when it looks as though they are representing another country before America, we hope they are not. U. S. politicians exhibit scruples, morals, and ethics that serve as a model for our citizens and the rest of the world, too. Our government creates exorbitant budgets, and the bill is paid by taxes from citizens in order to make America a better place for her people. That is it in a nutshell. We need to spend more at home and less abroad. Could it be any more obvious? It is not protectionist—it is crucial. I am not a terribly religious man. However, I do believe that God helps those who help themselves. We need to do that now.

Freedom, capitalism, and democracy sometimes need controls and structure to stay on track.

Chapter 4:
Be Controlled, You Socialist Pig

Americans have to learn how to help themselves again without fighting wars about obsolete fuel technologies that feed terrorism or fighting each other and creating further polarization. We all really want the same things—health, wealth, and happiness for everyone in the world. I am not a socialist, but concepts that divide us are the root of all evil. Competition is not divisive. It can be very healthy.

It would be much better if there were a standardized model of healthcare benefits similar to Medicare, one plan for everyone, single-payer, a health plan that everyone understood. Maybe the new system will emphasize preventive care and allow euthanasia in the case of the terminally ill or dying elderly? That concept has been ignored since the beginning of time.

Americans have very high expectations of our medical system. We should and doctors should.

We need to give the provider side the opportunity to deliver better outcomes with evidence-based standardized accountability for doctors, hospitals, and other care providers.

It is despicable that insurance companies have divided the risk pool of healthy Americans for profit. Providers need to be at risk and earn more dollars by keeping us well. Prevention makes healthcare costs go down. Internal medicine is the key—not as gatekeepers, but as active participants in their patients' health.

Do you think the CEOs of America's largest health insurers should have pocketed hundreds of million dollars over the past ten years? Does that sound reasonable considering the industry and its cost problems? Health insurance companies have laid off tens of thousands of employees lately. Social responsibility was never their forte.

Spreading the risk of health coverage over the entire population for one single-payer would definitely cost less. Is that universal? Yes and no. Instead of profits creating a surplus for more care when necessary, let's give it to greedy and incompetent executives. That has been the current theory. When you add in the savings from monopolistic buying advantages over the private sector, electronic health records and evidence-based medical practice, we may realize more than a 50 percent savings on the current system. That is right. When it comes to healthcare, the government should be allowed to negotiate the price. There are some limitations that do not disturb what is beautiful about the free market model of business in our democracy. The government doesn't have to abandon the free market culture in healthcare. They have to embrace what works and destroy what does not. It is a fine balance that we can have.

We should all be afraid and proceed with caution. However, the future alternatives are deadly. The current consumer-driven model of health insurance is the next financial fatality to shake our American foundation.

Remember, the more confused you are, the easier it is to take advantage of you in business. Yes, that is immoral and unethical. Sound familiar? That's what we have. Pigs. Monopolies are pigs.

Insurance is a necessary business in the world and plays an important role in all societies throughout the world. Insurance and healthcare could maintain some type of relationship from a supplemental standpoint. Risk-takers can be justifiably good for America and everyone else. For example, you are glad when you are well protected through insurance—especially when something goes wrong and your insurance company is there to pick up the pieces. Unfortunately, it comes at too high a price for healthcare, and you never know what they may or may not pay for.

Do not forget that insurance in healthcare—whether for profit or not—is poorly managed due to high costs of administration. It is too focused on profit instead of care—which is not their business in the first place. Even not for profit can mean profits when runaway general and administrative expenses are absorbed by poorly run insurance companies with extremely well-compensated executives.

When health insurance companies took control of healthcare away from providers, they were building their own profit machine.

Insurance company greed built its own coffin with respect to healthcare in America.

Health insurance companies have compromised the practice

of medicine and stunted the growth of more innovative means of protection.

Health insurance companies would do almost anything for healthcare delivery to be the single largest component of gross domestic product in America. We are headed down that road.

The current employer-sponsored model of providing healthcare protection is becoming an overwhelming administrative burden to companies. Managing the health of employees through the employer-sponsored model of insurance will break the backs of corporations legally and financially. It is pretty scary to hear a Fortune 500 CEO who knows that if he or she can somehow unload the beast of burden that benefits have become, their company would somehow welcome it, and everyone could win together. After all, human resource executives are dependent upon consultants and brokers because they can't be experts in everything.

This horrific credit crunch means there is no better time than now for America to take action. I am that consultant … what am I going to do? I am going to reinvent myself at fifty years old. That is right. The new healthcare tax will look cheap compared to the actual cost of premiums for health insurance protection in the near future. There are many lines of taxes that can be applied and slated for healthcare. I have so many ideas for accomplishing this.

Can we really afford this stupidity anymore?

Actual healthcare expenses are substantially outpacing both inflation and wages, which is killing us economically. America is going to experience much higher inflation due to our current 2009 economic crisis. The cost of medical advances, the advancement of pharmaceuticals we all crave when we get sick, and the current model of care delivery will cripple us financially—unless we act now.

Cost must be addressed fairly.

We can fix the healthcare system and pay for the benefits through appropriate use of taxes. Americans don't need more taxes—maybe on the ultra greedy rich and powerful—but America must start spending our tax revenues wisely. We need tax codes that penalize the industries that are hurting Americans' healthcare. It is not about how much money someone makes fairly—it is about whether or not there is any value added. There have to be consequences for the actions of irresponsible companies and their leaders with ungodly power. America needs simplified flat taxes that are fair to the common man and that take the new class of ultrarich into consideration. America is awaiting a new tax system that is fair and incorporates the challenges of absorbing the risk taken by the current health insurance company monopolies into consideration.

There are other things to consider in addition to catastrophic financial protection from medical problems. The healthcare system needs to be fixed from the inside out. It involves a lot more work than our grid locked, polarized system of government seems to be capable of accomplishing. Are they capable? Of course! President Obama has the leadership qualities to accomplish the mission. Remember that the ethics and morals of our government elected officials should be the mentor and model for how Americans should live their own lives. Companies and their management are behaving just like the government, which is why we have these economic troubles to begin with. Where is our fiscal responsibility? Does the government spend more than it takes in? Moral fiber and ethics ... do these ring a bell, Congressman? Now where will this stimulus package lead us?

Should America continue the mistake of punishing those in need while rewarding those in power—at the expense of her people's future? We are in very precarious times.

Chapter 5:
The Future of Healthcare.
Am I Touching You?

Why not mandate health insurance for all Americans? What a great idea. Now what? Just out of curiosity, why would you want to do that anyway? Because that will help the insurance companies continue to make record profits and allow their CEOs to steal from their policyholders and providers!

Mandating health insurance forces all Americans to be responsible. Where does the government get the nerve? American taxpayers provide their salaries. Have they been responsible with their decision-making? That is not protecting Americans. The government needs to be responsible and help Americans help themselves. Freedom did not get us in this mess. Leading by example will get us out of this mess. Do the right thing.

Americans need to buy into self-improvement and the good health movement. It is not going to happen from insurance, pharmaceutical, medical device and supply company advertising. Get those brainwashing exploiters off the air.

Congress overspends with money that is not rightfully theirs and that same perverse thinking has spilled over to the private sector at a huge cost to our citizens. It is a mentality that is corruptive and corrosive. At a depressing moment in financial history, we have to make the best decisions.

Do you think that mandating health insurance for all Americans will lower costs? It could on a per capita basis if done properly.

How will it help the system? It won't! A health mandate is not the answer as they found out in Massachusetts. Senator Kennedy's heart was in the right place. In his honor, Congress will fulfill his dream to overhaul the US healthcare system..

The medical system needs to be fixed. Then—and only then—will every American citizen and visitor to our country be able to afford medical care when necessary—anywhere in America. Rural needs are always difficult to respond to. That is the way it is in every healthcare system including our current one. At least America has excellent access through transportation. This could be another infrastructure earthquake in the making.

Healthcare should have become a more competitive business. Instead, over the past twenty years, the private sector has sucked the juice out of it, and the health insurance business has become less competitive and monopolistic. Healthcare has become controlled by insurance. Most states have *one* dominant health insurance carrier. What kind of competition is that? Just ask your state attorney general.

America has no choice. America needs to get the monopolies out of healthcare. There is only room for one solution. That is not socialized medicine, but if you understand the differences, you can help the United States to rebuild the healthcare system, constructively and in the best interests of all.

Private companies have not demonstrated the ethical leadership necessary to create innovative solutions to tomorrow's problems in healthcare. It takes the highest degree of integrity, ethics, and morals, which are usually not found when profit is your primary motive. Try laying off more employees while CEOs take home huge bonuses. Free markets?

I own an insurance agency, which sells health insurance to Employers and individuals. I consult physicians and negotiate contracts with health insurance carriers on their behalf for better reimbursement. I hear a lot of complaints. I service my group health insurance clients, as best as I can. There have been numerous times where I felt compelled and forced to challenge health insurance company legal departments. When health insurance companies don't honor their contracts, I advocate on my client's behalf. Do you know who complains the most? I only service insured employers who offer their employees group health insurance along with other employee benefits. We also do business with individuals in a vast array of insurance products. We only represent the largest and highest rated health insurance companies in the country. When they are wrong and my client is right, I fight them with intensity and passion. By learning the laws, I am able to argue on my client's behalf very effectively. I have numerous stories about fighting insurance companies and how to win. Is your broker helping you?

America needs to declare a state of national emergency for its healthcare system.

It is time to recognize what the manipulative, powerful enemies of change have done. In addition to the health insurance industry, this obviously applies to the banking, financial, and mortgage industries.

Don't lose focus of the real problem.

Mandate is defined by Webster's dictionary as "an authoritative command; especially: a formal order from a superior court or official to an inferior one."

So there you have it … another bad idea. Uncle Sam is now ordering us inferior ones around. Who works for whom? Where and how is your tax dollar being spent? Do you want some bureaucrat—who has numerous affordable choices of health coverage available to them—telling you that you must go and purchase protection? Is that your reality? That is all right … they won't be able to afford it for long.

We must level the playing field and remove the psychological burden on our citizens. Small businesses are getting murdered. That is bad for America. We need to create more jobs and increase the tax base. Healthcare is the answer. The only other choice is to have protection paid for by some other means. When any American citizen inevitably needs to utilize medical services, there is some money to pay for your health needs now that you did not protect yourself from catastrophic financial disaster to begin with. Maybe that makes the most sense. Catastrophic financial protection that is paid for through taxes after building up a system of reserves that counts on a government and a Congress that does not spend money it does not have. In other words, a government that always runs a balanced budget. Ingenious. It will be a decade before that happens again, sooner, I hope.

America wants her government's leadership to have the courage to walk the talk. Are all the human rights that we fight for around the world a bunch of hot air? Is it our security or our freedom that healthcare protects? Does healthcare protect our children or our leaders?

Mandating does not always create compliance.

What do we do when Americans start falling through the cracks in the system? Do we throw a sick American who did not contribute to the system for whatever their reasons "back on the street" or do we have a compassionate system that protects "human rights" and does the best we can within the means of our healthcare system? Do we help this poor slob? Do we put them in jail for not paying their bill? Do providers just write it off as bad debt? What kind of rhyme or reason or logic applies here?

How about getting them a job where training for the future is available? We can identify all Americans citizens through our new healthcare system and ferret out the illegal immigrants who do not pay taxes and send the money they earn here back to their countries where they belong unless they become legal citizens where they can pay taxes too. I don't think that is so difficult if we choose to help them and ourselves too.

I look to President Obama for this leadership. He is a very capable and well-educated man. Mandates need enforcement. How much is that going to cost? Who will decide the penalties of noncompliance and how will they be enforced? How much will that cost? What we have is an idea that has no foundation vested in the future except another profit motive that will set us further in debt. Hmmm. Smells like oil.

Every American knows that healthcare costs in this country are outrageous. Single-payer will lower costs in addition to many other excellent suggestions coming from our current panic mode.

The insurance law of large numbers will apply as we get the uninsured population into the system. We will be spreading their risk with premiums. Who should benefit from that? Should America and her citizens as a whole or should some monopolistic insurance and pharmaceutical companies benefit? History has a habit of repeating itself. This is the time to make history.

I find everything is in the semantics. Instead of the word mandate, maybe we should explain to Americans what this fight about the healthcare system really means and what is at stake for which stakeholders?

Insurance companies always win. They came over on the Mayflower with Lloyds of London. God bless them. They understand and take risk. They have their place in society. When you pay them for protection and you need them, they are there most of the time. That is our expectation. They can't always deliver due to poor management and unexpected genuine catastrophic disasters. However, they can plan for it and do the right thing.

Why all of the confusion in health insurance? Sadly, it is by design.

Where is the consumer's protection?

It is in the profit.

Mandating using the current healthcare system will simply serve as another very expensive Band-Aid that will punish the liberals who only wanted to do the right thing in the first place.

Healthcare isn't about liberals and conservatives or Democrats and Republicans—it is about human life and rights in America.

Americans are all red, white, and blue. We are all human beings. We all bleed red.

Healthcare should not be a privilege and mandating it will only mean some more people who can hardly afford coverage now will be forced to buy it—another bureaucratic blunder that we are becoming famous for in the rest of the world. Yes, America is having some issues that amount to no big deal if we make the right choices going forward. We have proven very resilient.

If you, Congress, want to mandate anything, then mandate healthcare services for all Americans as part of the new Bill of Human Rights in the Constitution. That is the new deal we need.

Through a constitutional amendment, healthcare can be the domain of the government like it is for Medicaid and Medicare.

We can do this and do it right. It is not socialistic or communistic. America will be doing what is right for her future. The health of American citizens is directly correlated to success as a twenty-first century competitor in the world. America needs this now.

There are so many savings that can be realized through a radically different healthcare system. Our new medical system will once again be the envy of the world. The United States is not like other countries that have socialized medicine. We have a lab or MRI center on every corner near any major city. Remember, we have better access to care than any country our size.

The government, as a single-payer, can be held accountable without profit in mind and with the best interests of Americans at hand. Take the profit out of healthcare by changing the incentives that currently permeate the healthcare system. Evolve to a single-payer system to remove the confusion and clutter for doctors and hospitals and other extensions of medical access. Let the healthcare system and its respective providers of care practice medicine as it is meant to. Remove the legal system barriers to better care. Mandate online health records and coordination of care for all Americans and we will emerge stronger and healthier.

There is only one major problem with single-payer. It may lead to socialized medicine. We will see and should see. As the free markets turn toward monopolies, it brings higher risks. The underwriting curve in health insurance is headed south for a period of ten years. Our population is aging as a nation. The level of fraud in healthcare is disgraceful. Sure, the insurance industry created tremendous overhead for doctors. The oversight of insurance companies in healthcare always perplexed me. What were they doing there in the first place? Oh yeah, the HMO Act of 1973. Was that a good thing or not? Good and bad. That is another story.

You want oversight … listen to this. Most doctors will not prescribe anything for you unless you come in and see them. However, insurance company medical directors seem to think it is okay to adhere to the corporate mission and make medical decisions for reimbursement regarding life and death situations and don't see the patient. They sit inside their little glass offices thinking of ways to increase profit and lower unnecessary care expenditures for their company.

If you want some marketing fraud, listen to all of the insurance company literature about special programs that address chronic disease. Overcoming resistance to change for Americans with chronic disease is a difficult challenge for all parties. So far, outcomes are hardly changing for the better. There must be more effective ways of helping Americans who will accept the help. What can we do as a single-payer that insurance companies won't do and how will it affect the bottom line?

There is no question that the U. S. healthcare system needs a cure of its own. We have a severe provider shortage—doctors, nurses, and a host of other supportive roles. There will be less specialty medicine, but it will become highly specialized. That will not make up for the coming deficit of physicians. How many plastic surgeons can there be? Don't get your hopes up because reality is that plastic surgery is not getting less expensive and your fancy-assed boob job and facelift will not come at a cost to other taxpayers. Pharmaceuticals are playing a more active role in healthcare and prevention sometimes. What can we do to halt runaway demand? Our health is not oil.

Free the American spirit by mandating a constitutional amendment to support the new healthcare system.

America cannot afford to mandate her citizens in an economic crisis. Besides you are wasting more money while the clock to disaster is ticking. Most in the know would say Americans with health insurance are already trapped due to forced migration by insurance companies. Plan design changes, from indemnity plans thru managed care plans to consumer-driven care plans and Health Savings Accounts. Insurance companies don't care. They never did. Their business is risk. Oh ... and big rewards at your expense. Unfortunately for them, it will come to an end with healthcare. They still win because the risk or underwriting cycle in healthcare is rounding the curve southbound toward a downward trend for the next 5–10 years at least due to America's aging population and several faulty strategies. Less profit for the insurance companies unless the respective State Insurance Departments grant their wishes for huge premium increases. It could also be a win for insurance companies if we fix the system from the inside out and they still maintain control. Watch out for some more plan migrations designed to make you think you are paying less. The reality is you will be paying so much more.

Cooperate and be a rat ... that is what they want.

As long as Americans are willing to flock from one flawed health insurance plan design to another, progress on cost in healthcare is doomed. Passing an unreasonable amount of cost sharing onto the sick while they are ill is really showing them that we care. Why not just throw your momma from the train?

Now that is a fine example of protecting human rights in America.

The Republicans suggested tax breaks to all Americans who purchase health coverage through Health Savings Accounts. Can I ask you something? Do you know that Americans have the lowest rate of savings ever since it has been measured? Do you really think when pension funds and banking institutions are failing and the false corporate promises of free healthcare for life to retirees is disappearing, that Health Savings Accounts are going to cure the ills of the healthcare system? Consumers are dangerous to themselves when directing their own care. The whole consumer driven model is dangerous.

Cost sharing through the use of your health savings account will not solve anything. It will not create competition for healthcare services because the measurements of quality have so much more developing to do in order to be effective. High deductibles may lower cost temporarily until what could have been prevented becomes a really expensive healthcare issue.

The Health Savings Account is an invention that some insurance company and banking company executives sold to the Bush administration. What a crock. The Health Savings Account movement is not working because it only addresses over utilization, which is not the core or major problem. It is another temporary fix with no longevity. They figure that if it costs more, you won't use it. An ounce of prevention is worth a pound of cure. Some insurance company executive must have thought, gee, if we stop them from going to the doctor, we can keep a larger percentage of the premium for ourselves.

Health Savings Accounts don't work or have anything to do with the current problems of our healthcare system. Health Savings Accounts make larger companies think they are lowering their costs. The employee can only see their contribution to the premium is lower—not what it means to their life if they get sick. Lower middle class to lower class folks depend on employer-sponsored health insurance—as do most of their higher compensated counterparts. Health insurance premiums have skyrocketed and many Americans—who need coverage and can afford it—can't get it because of medical underwriting requirements or preexisting conditions issues. Utilization is not the real problem. Legal cherry picking is the problem.

Cost is the most solvable problem in healthcare.

There are many other issues too. However, giving tax breaks to Americans who need their insurance premium money to buy groceries to eat will not solve the health insurance crisis in our country. The truth is that Health Savings Accounts equal big banking profits—not that I am against making a profit. Our banks need all the help that they can get, thanks to some mighty greedy gambling with your money. However, we are talking solutions and reform.

Health Savings Accounts simply adopt many of the same concepts that have helped to land the healthcare system in the current state of garbage. Our insurance companies were happy to see this development as their executives padded their pockets. It was a calculated risk that went sour for insurance companies. Healthcare should not be profit-motivated—it should be socially motivated in yes this capitalistic republic called the USA. I hate to use the "social" word because it is politically incorrect.

Don't be part of the problem … be part of the solution.

Health Savings Accounts plan designs which are attached to High Deductible Health Plans (HDHPs) create medical debt. Bankruptcy due to medical bills is rising at an alarming rate. The credit and collections scam is running rampant. Watch out.

Currently, American doctors and other providers typically only get paid for 70 percent of the services they deliver. Now with the growth of the Health Savings Accounts, medical debt is skyrocketing! That is not fair. You want to be paid when you work or provide a service.

This strategy is great timing amid our doctor and nursing shortage.

Are doctors going to be pleased or want to cooperate with positive change when they can't even get paid for doing their jobs?

The use of tax breaks and Health Savings Accounts is clearly a strategy that is doing more damage than good.

Consumer-driven care through the use of high deductibles may curb utilization trends for all of the wrong reasons.

The consumer-driven movement is an insurance company move—not a move by consumers. Somebody writes a book and all of a sudden, the Information Age is going to replace the need for a coordinated medical system. People with high deductibles continue to use crisis-oriented approaches to wellness. How does that fix the escalating problems associated with the cost of medical care? It does not. The lack of health information technology in healthcare practice is embarrassing.

Preventive utilization comes with education and the willingness of the insurance company to provide those benefits in exchange for premiums in the way of plan design and covered expenses. Insurance companies are grudgingly allowing for moderate amounts of preventive care expenditures while many doctors abuse them. There is no coordination of care and the limits on preventive care theoretically are based upon the same broken crisis-oriented healthcare system that we have now.

Consumer-driven care is an anecdote supplied by insurance companies. It does not work and will continue to erode the healthcare system.

The message insurance companies, Corporate America, and Congress needs to hear is "You can't brainwash us anymore." The American people are surprisingly resilient and getting stronger. We will force change upon the system with a concerted effort from the people of the United States—not the insurance, pharmaceutical, medical supply, or provider side of the industry. We will mobilize our power to create positive change. America can do much better. We should be ashamed of ourselves. Helping everyone else but ourselves is getting us in more trouble.

When is the government going to remove drug pushers from television advertising?

Pharmaceutical companies are pushing their drugs on TV as though American citizens and patients ought to tell our doctors what they should prescribe us. How perverse. Yeah ... when I went to see my doctor the other day, I told him I needed a prescription for oxycodone and marijuana. Seems my anxiety is overwhelming me. He said, "No problem, man."

Why go to the doctor at all if what we need is the message we see and relate to on TV from Big Pharma? Not only do all of these commercials sensationalize the potential lifestyle positives of the prescription drugs they are pushing, they downplay the side effects and dangerous combinations of drug interaction so the commercials leave you with a perceived need and no real education. After seeing those commercials, you go tell your doctor what you think you should be prescribed.

Shouldn't your doctor know which drug to prescribe?

When marketing becomes dangerous to our future needs as a

nation, we usually take some steps to prevent it from continuing. The same thing that was done with the tobacco industry advertising now needs to be applied to Big Pharma. How long are we going to wait? The taxes imposed on Big Tobacco should be imposed on Big Oil and that money should go directly to healthcare. That goes for fast foods, too. The obesity problem, which leads to dozens of expensive treatments, is promoted daily on television and we have made it the least expensive way to feed ourselves. America is a breeding ground for Type 2 diabetes from obesity. I remember when people went fishing to feed their families. Those taxes are supposed to go to healthcare.

Our use of prescription drugs is increasing at an alarming rate. It is alarming because many of these innovative pharmaceuticals save lives and prevent hospitalizations, which is how they justify their expense. Treatment in place of prevention is our approach to sickness. The expenses associated with this increase in utilization of prescription drugs are obscene by other advanced country's standards. Our reliance on Big Pharma to do the right thing is never going to be realized. Their marketing machines are part of the medical terror axis of evil that pollutes our citizen's minds through television advertising. America has its own medical terror network or axis of evil—and they even have good intentions. Maybe axis of evil is a little overstated. However, profit is still their primary motivator, which sounds fine in a capitalistic democracy—except when it hurts Americans more than it benefits them. If Big Pharma took all of its marketing money and put the money into reducing the cost of drugs in America, our healthcare system would not be as plagued and much needed innovative prescriptions could become affordable.

The world's pharmaceutical and bio-pharmaceutical companies' research are unlocking medical secrets and challenges to disease and illness that are helping humanity and ending common illnesses. Their place is a vitally important one. They deserve the financial rewards that capitalism affords them to a certain extent, but they are still part of the problem due to the cost of their products. Why are our own companies ripping us off? They get the protection at the cost of American lives. Patent protection for seven years is unreasonable. Advertising without any protection for Americans but the FDA is unconscionable. Americans are victims of their own desire for immediate gratification. We are an easy sell when it comes to our healthcare. Where are the health insurance industry and their cohort's sense of decency?

It has been suggested that we throw away employer-sponsored coverage. The problem is that some want to eliminate it for all of the wrong reasons. Americans have grown so dependent on their employers for health coverage that they often cannot retire due to their unaffordable health coverage needs. It keeps Americans at work. Americans under the age of sixty-five cannot afford to retire and pay the full premiums for healthcare coverage. Individual healthcare mandates will fail. Americans cannot afford them. Employers would welcome a 5. 5 percent tax to pay for benefits—given the right set of incentives. We are going about healthcare reform in the wrong ways. It is not to penalize; it is to reward most business.

What kind of human rights are we representing here in America, anyway?

The consumer-driven movement in healthcare is another smokescreen for plan design changes that involve more cost-shifting to you and me or more financial responsibility to burden the insured. Many large consulting houses typically survey large employers. The trends in their reported responses are largely company driven. Not everything you read is gospel. Sometimes questions lead to get the desired answers. Small businesses and entrepreneurs are getting murdered financially. They create jobs.

Those tricky monopolistic insurance company CEO pinheads are setting up more self-enriching guidelines for care. Why are they controlling the medical system? Because we were asleep at the wheel when we let them take risk and control reimbursement to providers.

The reality is that current trends in healthcare costs add up to a disaster for the future of America.

It has been estimated that healthcare expenditures will account for over 50 percent of gross domestic product in the year 2025 if we don't change our attitudes toward healthcare now. There is a way to manage this beast and keep the current healthcare crisis from overtaking our economy in less than twenty years.

Should individuals decide their own fates when it comes to healthcare?

Health is a personal responsibility, isn't it?

What if you are not born healthy?

With all of our emphasis on green, natural, healthy living, why are so many fast food restaurants mobbed with fat Americans stuffing their faces with unhealthy foods?

What if you have great financial stress and you develop substantial health problems?

We listen to pharmaceutical companies pushing their drugs on seniors and chronic disease sufferers every day on the television. I repeat, these advertisements should finally be banned from the air. Consumer-directed care is poison. We need a model of care that stresses prevention and education. It doesn't have to be transparent. It has to help and be a good value.

One health plan for all Americans will work and will be the best thing to happen to this country since the Declaration of Independence—not to mention the long-term savings and future health of Americans in protection of our freedom, democracy, and capitalism. Yes, capitalism. I should not have to defend it, but the greedy pinheads that care to argue are those that are either getting shafted or have too much already.

How can Americans, not doctors or clairvoyants, be expected to understand what particular medical services they need and how they are covered for them. Heck, if I had a crystal ball, I would have been an insurance or pharmaceutical company. Only, I wouldn't have stolen from those in need. Employers should be congratulated for sponsoring coverage for their employees. Large employers who self-insure and take the usual risks of an insurance company enjoy the control and savings that self-insuring can yield them. They are afraid of how a new system will affect their bottom line and their employees' job performance. The government must provide them with a clear incentive. More jobs that focus on core efforts and not human resource functions that simply revolve around healthcare benefits will mean greater profits and more Americans with career futures. What about healthcare coaches for everyone? How are we going to afford that? We can't afford not to.

What will happen if employees no longer need their employer for healthcare coverage? They will pay a tax that will be less expensive in the long run than managing the costs associated with administering the human resources necessary to handle health insurance.

No one knows, and yet it could create a huge economic explosion of productivity through creativity and innovation. When you free the human mind and spirit from constant financial burden and healthcare worry, the number one and two issues for Americans in the workplace today, great things usually follow. I am bullish on this concept. It works. We are America.

The healthcare system needs some major restructuring prior to the economics of change producing any significant effects. We can multi task and resolve many economic issues at once. Leadership is about making a positive difference in the majority of Americans' lives. It is time to execute the change.

If the United States enacts mandated insured individual coverage at the expense of employer-sponsored coverage, we simply continue the current death spiral of the current system.

You will remember the winners and losers of healthcare reform. They may never let us forget.

If the winners of reform are not all Americans, who do you think is winning?

When the winners manipulate the outcome, they think the outcome is already fate.

On one hand, we are critical of the government, Congress, and the president because we have a right to be. They work for us—the taxpaying citizens of this great country. On the other hand, as pitiful as Uncle Sam can be, when the majority of Americans begin to fight for justice within the healthcare system, a metamorphosis will begin. The private sector has its own agenda, which is profit at your expense. When Americans realize the trouble we are in and want healthcare services as a national right and understand the benefits of a One Plan System, they will get behind the agents that lead to constructive change.

Create a One Plan government-sponsored alternative while we work on fixing the system ills and let competition give the insurance companies a run for their money. Don't set us taxpayers up to be the insurer of last resort as we are for the uninsured and Wall Street.

Regulate those robbers of change—the health insurance companies. Modernize the inspection process so nothing falls through the cracks. Level the playing field and eliminate all insurance company medical underwriting and pre-existing conditions clauses before creating a government-sponsored alternative.

Maybe insurance companies will be able to stop the movement toward single-payer, but I sincerely doubt it. It is just a question of time and how well we transition to what could be the most significant positive thing to happen to America and her people since the New Deal. This is a financial grand slam for America.

Vote no to individual coverage and the elimination of employer-sponsored health insurance coverage until we figure out how to do the right things within the current medical system. It will buy us some time, but we must act quickly. Our economy demands it.

When we accomplish some of the advances that many other respected voices on healthcare are talking about, the private sector will have its last stand or learn how to do the right thing. The government will have the opportunity to show the great people of this nation what human rights are all about.

What are you counting on?

Who can you trust more?

I emphasize again that the private sector is focused on profit at your expense—under all circumstances. The difference is that the government works for the American people with no profit agenda. Our government can be fiscally responsible, and our citizens can maintain and even increase their economic stability.

The key to America's resurgence to economic prosperity is healthcare and protection from catastrophic disaster. Healthcare is where it is at—not Wall Street. How can you compare the returns of good health versus money? Just ask any sick rich person.

The Centers for Medicare and Medicaid Services run Washington-based social programs for seniors and the poor. Their administrative costs are reported to average only about 4 percent. If you run a company, then you know how remarkable it is. Health insurance company costs average as much as ten times that of Medicare. They pay for it by ripping us off. Of course, the states control and dictate variations in the Medicaid program, which is part of the reason why it is so messed up. These programs were created by LBJ in the sixties and still work extremely well—even when you consider our aging population, medical advances, and what these programs were designed for.

Are our elected officials asleep at the wheel? Who could ever believe that?

We all get ripped off when our tax money gets spent in ways that are not in the interests of the majority. Capitalism can bring out both the best and worst in society. Healthcare is a right. Unfortunately, good health cannot be guaranteed for all.

Employers are critical to the reform movement in the healthcare system and must be assured that reform will be good for them, too.

Most employees want more control of their healthcare dollar because they have been led to believe that is what is missing. American workers really want choice. Americans want more preventive care, alternative care coverage, and ways to customize healthcare coverage. Additional customization to a One Plan Model can be created through gap plans that complement the core standardized single-payer medical plan.

Remember that the current rhetoric of reform is all brainwashing to keep the private sector in the profitable healthcare business at your expense. Customizing coverage could be an adjunct to the core medical coverage that a single-payer system would bring to the table at significant administrative savings—close to 50 percent of every coverage dollar. Insurance companies could still provide additional protection similar to Medicare gap plans. Every American would win. What is wrong with that? Powerful stakeholders don't like to lose—that is what's wrong. They want to control the outcome.

So, who are you going to trust more—the private sector of insurance companies who screwed everything up to begin with or the government? The U.S. government created Medicare. Any American who is thinking about healthcare and planning retirement at some point in time sure hopes Medicare is around for them too.

Don't fall for those smart, yet unconvincing arguments that socialized medicine is terrible all over the world. Statistics tell a completely different story. However, the United States does things better and differently than the rest of the world. Don't lose confidence in America's healthcare future. If Canada had our economy and medical infrastructure, socialized medicine would look completely different there. Our economy is in a constant state of change. Given our current economic difficulties, our economy will still prove the most resilient in the world.

"Universal Government-Run and Sponsored Health Insurance Protection Creates Huge Economic Expansion Opportunity for Business" will be the headline that captures world respect.

If you want to help small business create more jobs, then help us. Healthcare is the next boom in America. Be part of it. Be healthy.

Imagine as a CFO, not having to plan or budget for the unpredictable spiraling costs of employee benefits. Your company will keep more profits and not have competitive worries associated with benefits. Sure, all of us will pay more taxes and not have the tax write offs for the cost of benefits. The relief from paying monthly core benefits premiums will pave the way toward Corporate America becoming more competitive and productive. A change of focus in the practice of healthcare toward preventive care and wellness will create more satisfied, productive, and effective workers—not to mention a lot more jobs.

By embracing single-payer One Plan healthcare, America will get back to competing for market share based on the quality and price of our products. Lower healthcare costs will be coming at just the right time in our history.

Do you know that some of America's healthcare executives have taken home as much as $150 million per year? If I do my math correctly, that amount would create 2,000 jobs at $75,000 per year for Americans who need the work, have the expertise, and are more productive than the average employee. The service is terrible at health insurance companies because no one understands anything and they have eliminated tons of jobs whose salaries are now being funneled to the highest paid executives. That extra money is *not* going toward care for patients who need the benefits. Is that fair? Immoral losers.

Can you imagine a world that buys our manufactured products in addition to our services? Apparently, not.

An American single-payer healthcare system will send our financial markets through the roof. America needs this now! If not, Depression-like financial times will continue for a decade. With single-payer, America will be booming.

Employees can be treated more fairly with little chance of health discrimination. HIPAA privacy and confidentiality issues have created more problems than good. With single-payer, the administrative hassles—not to mention the enormous savings—will all be protected in one place. America can be price competitive and industry will prosper. However, before we make that move, understand that our tax system also needs to be overhauled and simplified with less room for innovative tax-avoidance strategies that tax code experts advise their extremely wealthy clients of. Extremely wealthy means having a net worth of $10 million or more. Yes, if you can pay your bills, some might consider that extremely lucky, but that is not wealthy in America. *It shouldn't be a privilege to earn a living.* Are we not the land of opportunity? When you earn more than the average person does, you are doing well. At $5 million a year, you are extremely privileged. Today there are almost one million Americans that are worth more than $50 million. There are close to one thousand billionaires, worldwide.

Are the political parties focusing on America's future or just going through the motions?

America may not have another opportunity to fix our exhausted medical system. Keep ignoring this problem, and dream on that everything is okay. It is not. Why is there such polarization in this country? Because most of us realize that our Congress lost touch with what ails us as a nation. Health insurance reform needs to be dealt with now. Americans need the medical system to change for the better, now. What are we waiting for?

Insurance companies rule the healthcare system. The government protects Americans from those risk-takers with mandates that govern the way they conduct business. What a crock of bull. Our government has set a poor example. There is no excuse for not knowing the difference between right and wrong. We are lackadaisical.

Congress rarely responds in advance to any problems we encounter as a nation. I am encouraged by the recent passing of the Genetic Information Act. Our global future is very competitive, and we have a wonderful opportunity that will pass us by given the forces of nature or big business. Insurance companies have a very poor track record as medical advances became more available and utilization trends increased. Yet, that is not the only place where the problem lies. We have to reverse our thinking on healthcare. Insurance companies have become more influential than the medical profession itself. If medicine is to be governed, then it should be done prudently. Switching plan designs and calling it a movement every ten years is not working when profit still drives the thinking.

How do Americans unselfishly help transition the healthcare system into the best, most effective, and most efficient system in the world?

Insurance companies and large self-insured employers are spending too much time finding ways to avoid taxes and paying claims instead of innovating and doing the right thing.

Average Americans look at all of Corporate America with contempt—especially Big Insurance and Big Pharma.

It is sad that a few bad eggs are affecting the way Americans look at the private sector leadership. America and our democracy stand for entrepreneurial endeavors and innovations that lead the world in so many ways. We are capitalists, but are we realists? We are a generous people, gifted in so many ways. For the majority of Americans, taking back control of your destiny will be the biggest challenge of our lives. Free the American spirit and fight to make healthcare part of our constitutional rights.

Chapter 6:
Cost Containment
Challenges

Why deal with the medical system cost issue when Americans need our lame-duck Congress the most? Thanks to them, we are at our most desperate financial moment in modern history.

Medical costs come at you in so many different ways. Ever been sick?

You sure as hell don't want to be sick in America.

Our entire economy is designed to kick you when you are down. We don't have to be socialists or communists to help other countries that have no human rights. But here in America, it is a different story.

For decades, medical costs have been outpacing the rate of inflation. Americans have great expectations from their healthcare system. Medical advances, insurance, pharmaceutical, and medical device companies—all of us want to make money. So do hospitals, doctors, and other providers. They have every right to make good money. They are well educated, responsible, and—for the most part—committed to excellence.

Commitment to excellence in American medicine doesn't always show up for the party.

We may know that medicine is an inexact science, but it can still be held to the highest standards. Corporations have removed the more social aspect of healthcare from our lives. Accountability for excellence should be at the top of every corporate goal. Unchecked expectations have gotten lost in the dust, and there are so many medical errors. Whether it is rates of readmission, morbidity rates, and mortality rates, we all want to stay out of medical institutions like hospitals—even if we need one. If you have been there or seen someone you love get care, ideally the outcome was pleasing.

Institutions and providers should be held accountable for outcomes. Using best practice guidelines through an evidence-based medical culture will elevate medicine in the United States to a new level, especially when combined with electronic medical records and other advancements. According to several studies at Dartmouth, the efficacy of some overutilized medical advances are questionable. Many American states, towns, and cities are consistently outside of the level of acceptability when it comes to cost and medical necessity of certain procedures. Reducing cost could mean better care and greater longevity.

The cost of medicine and whether healthcare is a right stands as a philosophical issue—not as the political one it has become.

Will we be violating the principles of democracy on which

our country was founded by expanding healthcare to the entire population?

Is standardizing benefits—so everyone can understand what they have—such a bad thing?

Someday, providers and billing services will even understand the medical reimbursement system if they only have to deal with one single-payer.

If Wal-Mart can sell prescriptions cheaper than your health insurance co-pay is, doesn't that tell you something?

Money pays for healthcare services—whether it comes in the form of taxes or income used to pay premiums for protection from financial catastrophe. Few Americans truly understand how their insurance works. Cost can be controlled through efficiencies and modern technology. Our political and legal system spends so much time over analyzing everything that they have analysis paralysis, inertia, or whatever you want to call it. If the United States wants it citizens to enjoy a better standard of living that freedom and democracy affords, we need to get in shape in this world of global competitiveness.

So, how do you deal with cost issues in the medical system? I can tell you one way you don't deal with cost issues and that is to let monopolies rule the game abusing their power to get what they want at the expense of the people they are supposed to represent. The only way the government can protect the people of American from runaway costs associated with medical care is to declare war on medical terrorism.

All Americans must do their part in the reform of the healthcare system. Here is some good news about reducing the cost of medicine.

Coordinating care in the new system through a cradle-to-grave preventive approach to medicine combined with technological and medical advances will save a lot of money. When we exercise, go green and organic, stop smoking and eating garbage, we will save money.

America can mitigate the cost issue by addressing our future positively. Where will we be as a people twenty-five years or one hundred years from now? Sure, defense of our freedom at any cost is part of America and our history. The way things are going, we may not have to worry about that. We are all headed for being baked by nukes because of all of the hostility in the world.

The cost issue in healthcare is about making a few perceived sacrifices. Reality is somewhat different. There are a plethora of funds flowing throughout the healthcare industry. Freeze the funds at this moment in history. We can achieve better outcomes at a significantly lower cost by injecting these suggested changes into the healthcare system.

Reimbursement incentives have to change. A crisis-oriented, procedure-driven medical system was always doomed for failure. The answer is painful at first. Change is difficult to accept when you take what you have for granted. When you buy into the fact that it is crucially necessary, you will embrace the change.

Transparency is nonsense ... where did they come up with this curve ball? The insurance company contracted price versus a private uninsured payer is vastly different. The insurance companies have buying power, which is why physicians band together into groups for some leverage on reimbursement negotiations.

Now that insurance companies will publish their reimbursement rates to doctors, will everything get better? No way. It will possibly blow up in everyone's faces, too. The entire reimbursement system in and around medicine needs to be revamped. It is not that providers make too much—or too little—money. It is what they get paid for. Fees do not need to be negotiated. They need to reflect the quality changes and future of our healthcare system. Single-payer will only be part of what straightens out our newly reengineered reimbursement system. We need to shore up the levees quickly or the quality of our medical system will continue to deteriorate. There are many new tools available to help the system perform at its very best.

The transparency theory assumes that it is helpful to know about a doctor's compensation for services rendered.

Hell, we can't afford pretty much anything they want to charge. Most people do not know much when they see a doctor—except that they are ill. After we see the doctor, we do not know what is written into their charts about the diagnoses or whether the prognosis is correct or not. Americans know nothing about acute, severe healthcare situations, except that they need care and have every reason to hope that the integrity of the medical system maintains its commitment to excellence. Having quality measures and other information could be useful, but it is not going to fix anything. Transparency tied to quality data could create some competition based upon unbiased and accurate data collection and interpretation.

The security Americans enjoy about our healthcare system will get better with time, but it has nothing to do with knowing what one particular doctor charges versus another one. It is easy to find that out anyway if you have some medical codes and do the research. Yes, transparency is tied to medical codes that underscore the entire reimbursement system to providers of care. Common Procedure Terminology or CPT codes are how physicians bill. Procedure-driven, utilization-laden, crisis-oriented medicine needs to change. We need to change how we pay doctors, hospitals, labs, pharmaceutical companies, and medical supply companies. Most reimbursement in and around the medical field is determined by insurance companies who are taking the risk and are responsible for reimbursement after receiving a premium in trade for protection from medical bills. It can happen—but will it?

Here is the perverse thing. The government paid to have a fair, reasonable, and responsible reimbursement system for providers developed for Medicare and Medicaid. Insurance companies have the talent to create a financial spread and to pay doctors less than that scale—which is subsidized by the government reimbursement system—to make an exorbitant profit. That causes the citizens to especially subsidize the uninsured at rip-off reimbursement rates created in providers' dreams.

The whole thing is crazy. Simplicity, quality through technology, and evidence-based care embraces all forms and aspects of treatment are the medicine America's healthcare system needs—not transparency.

As long as there is profit in healthcare, the patient's interests will always come second.

However, the truth goes beyond the obvious. While you think the medical system may be trying to save you, remember that the road to hell is paved with good intensions. For instance, when the elderly experience some sort of questionable procedure that could save their life for a few more months or years, the exorbitant amount of money spent goes unnoticed. It is spent because your loved ones expect you to look out for their best interests in the event they are not healthy enough to make that decision for themselves. Are we advocating the right thing?

You are forced to make medical decisions for your loved one—a new role as a healthcare advocate of some kind. Does it make you feel better to know that you are being placated by the amount of medical services they receive to help you, the relatives, accept their demise? Just look at the medical care that Americans receive during the last six months of life. Our medical system thrives at the cost of taxpayer dollars and our crisis-oriented approach to medicine. A small amount of providers really think of the quality of life for the elderly patient. Many well-intentioned providers are too busy practicing expensive and unnecessary medicine to their financial advantage to be truly concerned about the patient's quality of life.

Americans are immature, overly emotional, and sensitive about death. We have been led to believe that medicine at any cost makes sense. America needs to stop fooling itself about our healthcare system. When miracles happen, we are all especially grateful. However, too many elderly people—who are saved medically—end up suffering out their remaining days or years. Some are financially broke and in some form of a nursing home. Family stress runs very high in these situations. What is the quality of life for these seniors who are saved? The justification is that every situation is different. Does any doctor care? Do loving relatives care or is it their emotions that keep them from doing the right thing?

In spite of living wills, do-not-resuscitate orders, and other forms of personal protection, patients—especially seniors—are all just numbers. As long as the government (U. S. taxpayer money) is willing to pay (Medicare and Medicaid), the healthcare system will continue to reap undeserved compensation. In many ways, America's healthcare system has the attributes of the most dynamic and sophisticated medical delivery system in the world. We have always led the rest of the world in medical innovation. However, the overwhelming majority of Americans feel that the system needs change.

Medical errors, high morbidity rates, wasteful and unnecessary procedures, and a general lack of caring have invaded America's healthcare system.

The reality is that demand for medical services is running at an all-time high. Inflation rates are out of control. America is in the midst of a severe doctor and nursing shortage. Doctors are sick of being screwed financially and being told how to practice medicine by insurance companies. The health insurance underwriting cycle is beginning a downward trend. It is too bad that such well-compensated executives were so busy taking money away from the table that was meant for care.

The opportunity for insurance companies in the healthcare market is changing. Standardized plans, like Medicare and gap plans offer additional coverage to those Americans who care to purchase more healthcare coverage than Medicare. The single-payer national healthcare plan that every American will enjoy by 2020 can put us back on track.

Proposed changes to the healthcare system can be accomplished despite our economic issues. An article I read stated that health insurance premiums will double by 2017, but it does not tell the whole story. Most health insurance takes age into consideration. By 2017, those reading this realize that they will be nine years older. That means their premiums could easily be triple what they are today.

The war on medical terrorism must begin now.

Declare war on medical terrorism and be part of the fight. A single-payer system comprised of standardized plans or One Plan—evidence-based medicine that include best practices guidelines and incentives based upon quality-of-life measures that stem from preventive cradle-to-grave care—are the only answer. The system has more than enough money to pay for all necessary care—even for the uninsured. Yes, some difficult choices and limits must be drawn. There is so much money wasted in the medical system that America should be embarrassed by allowing private industry to abuse its own people down the devilish path of greed.

Isn't America a peace-loving, human rights-driven country? Instead of having social values that will work well in our democracy, we are choosing to ignore our needs at a huge price. It looks like Big Government, but single-payer will be a simplification of a complicated issue. It will protect all citizens and lower stress for our most valuable asset. . . our health. Americans with chronic illnesses, which still account for the majority of healthcare expenses, can be managed in ways that will lower costs and improve the quality of life for those individuals who develop or are born with those conditions and at a much lower cost.

Remember that it can happen to you.

When you eliminate profit-driven motives and actually get down to what is necessary, there is more than enough money to go around in our healthcare system. What will inefficient hospitals or other providers do when they can't bill the government for the uninsured who receive care at whatever price providers want to charge and receive tremendous tax write-offs for uncompensated services?

A single-payer system that insures all Americans at some standardized benefit level should have happened several decades ago.

This isn't about capitalism—it is about human life and human rights.

What kind of democracy doesn't even protect the human rights of its own citizens?

I will tell you who … America.

That is why we have no nationalized healthcare system. Why does the rest of the world look at healthcare so differently from Americans? From a healthcare and financial standpoint, America is doing poorly in almost every area of healthcare. Healthcare costs are on the rise around the globe. Different systems throughout the world face their own cost and quality issues.

Our healthcare system must emerge from reform and evolve into a much more efficient, cost-effective, uniquely coordinated care system that covers all Americans while maintaining the most attractive aspects of the system that insured Americans benefit from today.

By the way, I have been in the insurance industry since 1990. I was first licensed in 1985. Coverage guidelines must be established with cost in mind—combined with the best interests of the patients who need and utilize those medical services. The time for change is now. Declare war on medical terrorism. Change has to come and soon. Ignorance may be bliss, but it will catch up to you. Just look at our current state of affairs and the lack of confidence Americans have in the future of healthcare in America. Look at the 2008 presidential elections. President Harry Truman had an interest in a single-payer system in 1948, only to get struck down by the likes of the AMA and their elitist powerful friends. President Richard Nixon said America must not be dependent on foreign oil as an energy source in 1973. Now look at America's dependence on foreign oil. One can only avoid the inevitable for so long.

Change is accomplished when you keep demanding it and take back power from corrupt, greedy, and selfish people who call themselves leaders. They are managers of the way things are, not leaders with a vision of the way things should be. These supposed leaders are self-serving, brutal, and feel above the law. How tolerant have Americans become? Are we complacent? Are we competitive?

What is the government doing to make things better for you?

Chapter 7:
Where Do We Go from Here?

If Americans want lower healthcare costs and lower payments for the equivalence of some form of broad protection, Americans must participate in the change.

With just the obvious changes that are being recommended outside of my recommendations, we will notice significant differences in the way medicine is practiced. When we incorporate hard-to-accept changes to the system, costs stabilize and can be reduced as our statistical competitiveness in healthcare improves. It will all happen when we are ready; as a country and as united citizens, we demand change.

America must deal with the overwhelming demand and stress our citizens and noncitizens are putting on the U. S. healthcare system. Most Americans have health insurance, pay part of the premium, and share in the costs of the care. The majority of America is unfamiliar with their health plans and often gets confused and no reimbursement when they need the protection the insurance is supposed to afford them.

In a crisis, America always has a short-term solution.

The insurance companies are screwing around with plan designs and sharing censored information with their members while the government decides whether or not to punish them.

What can we do?

Most Americans feel that the tax system is too lenient on the rich. Rich bastards—let's steal all their money and give it to the poor. There are no more Robin Hoods, and life is not a fairy tale. Go out there and reinvent yourself. Are the poor not so poor and just healthy, smart, and unmotivated freeloaders who are gaming the system we built to help Americans in need? We need to define what is financially rich to start with. Naturally, those of us who are not wealthy have a tendency to expect more from those who are more fortunate by whatever means. I have to say that because there are a lot of inequities that bring about wealth in America. That is just the way it is.

When I was growing up, a million dollars was considered extremely wealthy. It would be nice to save or to earn a million dollars, even today. Most Americans will never reach that earnings level and certainly will have trouble accumulating a million dollars given the economy, our issues, the lack of savings rate, and our habitual spending. So, what is rich? One million dollars is not. Ten million sure as hell is. There are so many billionaires it is hard to believe. Good for them. I hope they are healthy and happy. Then, they are truly gifted. I define rich as having a wonderful family, spirituality, and my health. Everything else is extra.

Too much focus on money and not enough on health is bad for you.

If you are doing the best you can and are gifted with abilities that the average person does not have, you may be earning what others consider excessive. Too bad. It is the opportunity that capitalism offers us. We should admire any American citizen who earns and contributes fairly to the economic well being of America and themselves first. The IRS should be abolished and an actively policed flat tax should be applied to income brackets that fall above a realistic poverty level income. America should revamp healthcare and stamp out poverty. That is the least we should get accomplished.

The entire government should be reorganized with the next hundred years in mind. Every crisis bears an excellent opportunity. Cash businesses and illegal businesses must be monitored. What will the new tax system mean to the economy? The means by which executives accumulate wealth is largely through stock options where the long-term gains tax of 15 percent applies. What a great deal. When any American earns in excess of $25 million in one year, from whatever means, there has to be a special Alternative Minimum Tax applied to their income in increments that are extraordinary uncommon to the average American. Otherwise, the inequities of wealth will continue to evaporate the American middle class. The ultra rich are not trickling down squat, economically. Yet, when it comes to healthcare they are privileged because they can afford any treatments.

Trickle down economics is history. The benefits of that thinking disappeared more than twenty years ago. Facts show the trend is bad. Greed has set policy—not what is right and fair. A substantial amount of middle- and upper-middle-class taxpayers are not wealthy, but do earn between $100,000 and $500,000 per year. That is a lot of money, but it is not the real problem. They pay plenty of taxes versus their income. The majority of them pay for health insurance. We simply spend too much on the wrong things. Just think about what we could have done with the money we spent in Iraq!

However, America has established a wealthy and even an ultra-wealthy class of earners and accumulators who have paid very little taxes on their earnings. They are even beyond the upper class whose annual earnings are between $1 million and $5 million. Ultra-wealthy executives earn more than $5 million annually from a number of different means—including deferred income deals that set them up for life while their employees get screwed. Many high wage earners have an income in access of $100 million per year. That is obscene in healthcare and health insurance—it is *total* income from all sources, not a salary.

The estate tax is not fair and is double taxation. The real tax issue starts with earnings—not with accumulation after the proper taxes are applied and collected. Limiting capital gains taxes works up to a certain point. There is no risk in stock option grants—unless it is the only compensation being paid to an executive during a respectable period of time.

Do something about it, Congress.

The middle class as the silent majority became victims of inertia. Collectively they have the power to move markets, elect presidents, and other fantastic accomplishments. Yet, they are choosing to get sucked in by the laziness that is permeating our society. Now you may ask yourself, what does all of this have to do with our healthcare system? It all begins on a grassroots level. Our healthcare system has duped the tax system at the cost of American lives. Insurance companies and their partners own the U. S. government.

Now that Americans see the corruption that created havoc in our financial systems, maybe they will pay more attention to our free markets. Government employees with regulatory duties vital to our economic stability should be the best caliber of talent available and we should pay what the private sector pays them. Our officials are dumbfounded by the challenges of the private sector. You should also understand that somebody has to have the guts to enforce limits on care in the way that insurance companies do. It is not difficult when you are the one taking the risk to begin with. However, legally crafted underwriting and marketing programs that are designed to keep Americans from getting the care they need are wrong. Misleading and misrepresenting is a crime.

We are so busy doing business the old-fashioned way that creativity is being morphed into stupidity within the health insurance industry. It is unfortunately already too late. Someone should have allowed Ms. Clinton to get her plan in action. It was far from perfect, but her plan recognized issues that we are still struggling with a decade later. Put sacred cows out to pasture, and let's move on to the New America, which is a gentler, kinder, self-sufficient, and a stronger worldly ally that thinks of itself first. Our rights come first in America. The wake up call keeps ringing, and it is getting later and louder.

Single-payer healthcare equals American human rights.

Stop fighting for human rights? That would be anti-American.

We stopped here in America, but not around the rest of the world.

What a disgrace! Make healthcare a right by amending the Constitution and let the new healthcare system be the best it can be given the dire circumstances we are approaching.

It will take some time to reverse the current trends in medical costs, but the outlook could be astonishing.

It sounds cold when we are talking about healthcare and cost. We must make some difficult choices where everyone wins. That will be progress. There are definitely good times ahead if we make the right decisions and are conscious of the consequences of our actions. We have the data and lead the world in medical advances. The potential for improvements is fantastic.

Americans are already the most productive people on earth. Give America a break. Let's do what is right for our own people.

We are so busy helping other countries around the world with human rights issues that we forgot that our own people need the help of our government.

This change is not meant to be a handout to everyone who can afford or who currently has health insurance. It is not about de-motivating people who are dependent on the Medicaid system. It is not about being liberal or conservative, Democrat or Republican, secular or religious. Common sense and vision can only lead you to the same conclusion.

Any idiot can twist the realities of what is happening into a rationale that keeps the mistakes coming. We voted for change.

Create the 2012 New Deal on Healthcare, an amendment to the Constitution that provides the new system of healthcare to every citizen. After eliminating any form of underwriting or preexisting conditions clauses, the government-sponsored plan can be structured to compete with the insurance companies.

Competition will either bring out the best in the private sector or put them out of business.

Supplemental gap protection can still remain private, though the need for it will change drastically. America is ready for change. America must prepare for the future.

America's government must embrace the values that define our country, but not redefine the Constitution. Our Founding Fathers did not see this beast of burden coming.

Is President Obama proposing anything that your future grandchildren will be thankful for?

Is your president going to make sure that the medical advances we have access to can be utilized effectively and affordable to your children?

Make healthcare a right today.

Don't allow Americans to use Viagra, Cialis, and Levitra.

Why let us improve our lifestyles to reflect our wishes? Isn't that what freedom is all about?

By letting the insurance companies, the traditional Western-style medical system and lifestyle/genetic recklessness determine our health, are we really in control? No. We are out of control, plunging to our death through medical costs and dated philosophies. Is that what is so great about freedom in the area of healthcare? Because statistically, we rank significantly behind most developed nations in published healthcare quality measurements and pay so much more money than our global counterparts, it doesn't take a genius to figure out that something is fundamentally wrong with our healthcare system. We have to look at all of the players and yes, even our citizens and noncitizens, insured or uninsured are on the table. Americans are the utilizers of the U.S. healthcare system, and we must participate in the vital changes it needs, to improve it.

If we expect improvement from the folks we elect in public office, then we should expect it from ourselves.

Aren't you curious why 80 percent of the world uses alternative medicine as their primary means of treatment?

Is it all about money? What about your health? Take it for granted. After all you won't be sorry until you are sorry. Get the picture?

Organics are starting to make a real impact due to all of the new health conditions created by pesticides in fruits and vegetables imported from around the globe. What about the salmonella poisoning, too?

Exercise physiology is continuing to make a huge impact on Americans. Isn't it about time that Americans recognized the benefits of these discoveries in their healthcare system?

Green is just cool, fool—especially when it comes to fuel. What about the air you are breathing or the fact that there is a 50–50 chance of the North Pole having no ice next season? Times are changing. Get healthy and stay healthy. Don't become a victim. Get protection or you will be a victim. If you can't afford protection and don't qualify for public assistance, you are probably screwed.

Get behind the single-payer movement. Our economy desperately needs it. The medical society of providers who treat us, need it. You will be doing the right thing for America.

Support a constitutional amendment that guarantees healthcare to all.

Maybe socializing medicine is the answer. We already know the savings that will be realized from administrative relief through a single-payer system. Estimates are coming in at more than 25 percent savings.

Can we save even more money by rationing care? Yes. Rationing care is exactly what insurance companies do because all of their plans have limitations. Don't let the semantics get in the way of change.

We already have a socialized system that is combined with private industry—and it's broken. It is not the socialized part that is broken. Nobody is talking about taking away the freedom to choose. HMOs did that in another insurance company phenomenon. Low out-of-pocket costs lead to high utilization. Unfortunately, the wrong kind of utilization because of the way our system works. What about medical advances? America cannot afford unlimited healthcare within our current system of medical delivery.

Electronic health or medical records will have a major impact on wastefulness in the medical system. Provider response will be improved immensely from both a timing and quality perspective. That comes just in a nick of time; medical errors are rampant and getting more attention than what is good about our system.

Universal coverage is a home run for insurance companies. They'll see more profits at your expense. We can achieve universal coverage through vouchers where everyone signs up for a single-payer system. If you have an address where you can be found or a Social Security Number, you are already in. The problem will be identifying everyone else. That identification is good for America. We have so many illegal immigrants who need to be identified and helped to be on the road to citizenship. If the government wants to protect its citizens, we need to know who is living here. Profiling can help medical advances. The data is invaluable for the future of healthcare in the world.

Develop a fair way of compensating providers for their services, which every American can benefit from—not just a privileged few.

Lobbyists are paid big money to protect the profits of big business. They rule the game. The average consumer is lost in a maze of greed. Somebody needs to step up.

How many lobbyists represent the individual consumer who needs healthcare? Why resist change? I will tell you why. When the interests of big business clash with the interests of the majority, big business punishes democratic principles with its money and power. Democracy may have it pitfalls but are we united in the cause of better healthcare for all Americans. We all want to profit from our efforts here in America. A level playing field would help for rebuilding what is broken in our capitalism. Where is the representation of the common man? Remember when Harry Truman supported a socialized medical system that truly endorsed universal care? Now, sixty years later, we are struggling with the same concept. Just like energy, America waits until it is too late. We rarely have the vision to plan ahead. That takes leadership.

America embraces capitalism and should let profit drive all medical decisions. That is what we really need.

We have a system where the people paying for medical services have no rights. They say if you don't know what your rights are, you have none. Well, we all know the squeaky wheel gets the grease. Be persistent with your health insurance carrier. They can't win every battle. If you think you are truly right and being wronged, then get in touch with me. I can help you.

You see, Americans are not called the payers. The reason is that we pay insurance companies—the middleman—to take risk and to be the payers. Most insurance company legal departments can't even defend their positions when it comes to denying claims. The problem is that if you don't know what your healthcare rights are in their contract, then you basically have no representation. Seems like our politicians like it that way, doesn't it?

How many Americans in employer-sponsored plans really understand the legal issues when it comes to claims denial? Most brokers, agents, and consultants don't have the commitment and passion to bother understanding what it is they are selling.

There are thousands of coverage or plan variations offered by the top ten health insurance companies.

Is that choice or intentional confusion? The customized rationale fits in well with the right to choose.

Why does it have to be so complicated? If healthcare were simple, it would not be as profitable. What a rip off on America these self-serving CEO pigs created for themselves. It is deplorable that they are getting away with it. I ask you again, where is the value they creating? Is it just on Wall Street? Where is Congress in all of this? Due to ancient laws such as McCarron-Ferguson, allowing state governments to govern healthcare in varying degrees to address their different populations, Washington gave themselves reprieve. That was irresponsible. Healthcare in America is a federal matter—or better yet a national issue. It was never a state issue.

We are all red, white, and blue. Healthcare is a social issue and pretending that it is not ignores the needs of our citizens.

Reimbursement is laden with fraud. Who developed the current reimbursement scale? The government—with the help of some geniuses at Harvard University who developed a medical reimbursement system called RBRVS or Resource-based Relative Value Scale. RBRVS is a reimbursement system designed to reward doctors and other providers and suppliers that participate in the Medicare program delivering necessary services to those in need. As you now can see, the road to hell was paved with good intentions.

What you should know is that your insurance company negotiates well below the Medicare scale to reimburse providers of care in the private insurance plans we are paying so much for. Let me put that a different way. Did you know that your doctor—who treats your Medicare-eligible parents—gets a much higher reimbursement from Uncle Sam for the same medical services they may provide to you when reimbursed by your private insurance company? Insurance companies create a risk spread. It leads to higher profits when unfair underwriting practices and deceptive plan contracts are marketed. No wonder doctors hate insurance companies.

All health insurance should be guaranteed issue with no pre-existing conditions, clauses, or any underwriting of any kind.

I have to repeat this issue because without this change, progress on the other fronts will take years to accomplish. Health insurance or protection from financial disaster due to health issues should not be necessary and healthcare costs should be shared among all Americans. There should be more of a tax contribution from the more financially able. Why lie about it? That is reality and the right thing to do. That is democracy—not socialism. I am ashamed that I feel I have to defend my point of view from a political standpoint. Healthcare is a social issue and always will be.

In other words, the innovators of our current reimbursement system, started with a government contract and the insurance companies decided to abuse the physician community by negotiating reimbursement substantially below the scale. Do you understand why the government wants to take another look and perhaps lower the reimbursement levels for our public social programs? Obviously, if the private sector can negotiate below the uniform scale of reimbursement for our social programs, we are all paying too much. It is because the system was built on ancient principles tied to our crisis- and procedure-driven system. The wrong doctors are getting the wrong reimbursements. You know who you are.

The growth of well-financed specialty medicine took internal medicine out of the limelight. Now we are paying the price, literally. Coordinated care starts with your internist or pediatrician.

The real innovator to the future of our healthcare system will develop a revised reimbursement system that doesn't penalize providers for doing the right thing so some company can make a profit. All of the incentives have to change. The new reimbursement system will take into account all of the advances in all sectors related to healthcare.

Educating Americans on the cost of healthcare services is not a bad thing. They now call that transparency. Americans have a right to know what services cost. However, quality is rarely reflected in negotiated reimbursements with health insurance companies because the quality measurements that need to drive reimbursement are profit-driven instead of objectively arrived at. The result is that less care leads to more expensive care. Insurance companies can only hope you are off their books by then—so they don't have to pay your claims. The turnover from one insurance carrier to another is an expensive phenomenon.

Sometimes it is necessary to tear down something you build and to rebuild a better one. This is where America stands now. We need to build an entirely new foundation for our medical system that treats everyone in America equally. That is democracy, my friend. It can be realized if you support a human rights amendment to the Constitution for a single-payer, universal medical system designed to keep us well.

Now you can make some informed decisions and be part of the evolution of our new healthcare system.

Isn't it funny that all of the health insurance companies in America are scrambling to introduce new programs that identify chronic diseases, help manage them, and offer a small degree of preventive care protection? What is pitiful is that we have known for decades where the majority of healthcare dollars were headed and did nothing about it.

Isn't it funny that all of a sudden—when costs are out of control and health insurance profit forecasts are cycling downward—plan designs incorporate more cost-shifting to the consumer? That is because insurance is more about profit than protection.

Isn't it funny that the primary motivator in and around medicine has become profit and not achievement? Losers.

Isn't it funny that the same corporate CEOs who claim they are fixing the U. S. healthcare system created the problems to begin with? Disappointing would be an understatement.

Isn't it funny that hospital development around the United States is reaching an all-time high and solutions for healthcare costs are stuck in the same crisis-oriented system that exacerbated cost issues? When are we going to wake up? Teaching hospitals are experiencing a shortage of providers. What kind of future does that hold for our medical system? Who will staff all of these new facilities being built? What kind of care can baby boomers expect in the next twenty years?

Isn't it funny that America is experiencing an accelerating provider and nursing shortage and is challenged to create new solutions within our broken system of uncoordinated care? It would not be funny if you are sick and don't have the access to the right care. It is a privilege to be born with good health, but it's a smart decision to maintain good health.

Get yourself a healthcare advocate, ASAP. Doctors, spouses, children, relatives, and friends are all examples of healthcare advocates. Danielle, my wonderful wife, is my healthcare advocate. She's been trying to knock me off for years. That's because I'm worth more dead than alive. The truth is that I would be dead if she were not there as my health advocate when I needed one.

The key to true healthcare advocacy is timing and information.

Knowledge is the best tool for constructively organizing an advocacy plan for the potential victim of the system. Sometimes split-second decisions need to be made. This is not fun when you are dealing with the life or death of another person.

Advocacy is not medicine, but it consists of love and caring. When you get sick, who is there to make sure that the right medicine is being practiced? Who is there to make sure that you don't become another medical error statistic? Who is helping the patient make these life decisions?

Becoming a healthcare advocate is crucial at one time in particular. When your illness requires an acute in patient hospitalization or when you have a chronic illness that needs monitoring, you need an advocate. When you are being treated in-patient for more than seven days, your odds of getting well are dramatically decreased and correlate to in-patient time. Is there anyone that is coordinating your care? I doubt it.

We interact with so many doctors as our medical needs increase and there is no electronic coordination between them—except occasionally at the pharmacy. You need as many advocates as possible. There are too many treatment options and alternatives. There are good and bad diagnosticians. There are certain things that apply in each respective specialty. Multiple health issues need to be coordinated. Otherwise, each condition could exacerbate the other. Entrusting your life to a physician when you have no choice is one thing. But, most have a choice and do nothing about it. Try to coordinate your own care.

If you become sick, personally coordinating your own care becomes near impossible—depending upon your condition and the information that you need to have at your fingertips. Medicine is an inexact science, which is why advocates can be so important. Sometimes family history and genetic information is not shared with the providers. Lack of information has been known to cause a lot of medical errors. Americans should not have to be scared of personal identity theft or their personal health information or genetic history. Discrimination based upon health should be punishable as a criminal act. Still, in a perfect world, we need security and advocates who ensure that security. When it comes to an acute healthcare situation, there are times when you can't serve as your own advocate. Get a healthcare advocate—everyone needs one today. Start with research on the Internet. There are dozens of incredibly helpful sites.

Medical malpractice premiums are an ongoing issue for care providers. Premiums are expensive and provide little value but the protection they offer a provider even in the event of something uncontrollable or due to medical error. There has to be tort reform to punish originators of frivolous lawsuits and there must be a clear line drawn so consumers and their loved ones who access medical services know what to do when there is a real and definite problem. Lawmakers and regulators need to deal with repeat offenders on the provider side and not allow unsubstantiated lawsuits from the private side.

The current medical system reimbursement models are founded on principles of medicine that don't apply the same way anymore. There are foundations of science, and most of them are still pertinent to the highest levels of current medical thinking.

Medical and scientific advances, insurance companies, and drug companies have rendered the current reimbursement methodology obsolete.

There is no excuse for not changing the entire medical reimbursement system. There is so much information and technology at our fingertips waiting patiently to be imposed upon our medical system, which does whatever it takes to keep things the same. Change is at the forefront of this battle, and there are many high-profile, wealthy stakeholders that stand to lose big if the government endorses the right changes to the medical system.

The New Deal for the U. S. Medical System 2010 is a transition to single-payer, which will yield a great deal of relief to current and future generations. Americans will be able to concentrate on the economy, education, infrastructure, immigration, defense, global competition, and the sharing of resources with our allies. Believe it or not, restructuring our medical system will change the course of our history and pave the way toward newer innovative solutions that will allow the United States to once again enjoy world dominance in a number of peaceful, constructive ways to Americans and the rest of the world.

Americans are at a crucial point in history.

America and Congress … are you listening?

This is where capitalism meets democracy.

It could be said that capitalism is winning the war on democracy. Imagine the best medical system in the world—right here in the United States.

Is it your health and your life? Aren't they the same? Why is everyone trying to kill us? Your health insurance company doesn't want to pay your claims. The doctors or hospitals, labs or pharmaceutical companies or other drug dealers such as coffeehouses, soda, fast food establishments and insecticide companies just want your money. They don't care about the consequences of their actions.

Things have come a long way since the government has gotten involved in healthcare. For instance, just look at who is blaming whom over the spending or stimulus package or the over-spending in the medical economy. Yes, it is your lovely democratic and republican parties doing nothing good for America's future and just watching over their own interests. Our government does a great job of making healthcare coverage available to the poor or the elderly who qualify for it. There is no reason that the government cannot do the same for all Americans. Money is not the problem. It is psychological. No political party gets all of the credit, but the Democrats have their chance now. History is in the making.

Uncle Sam governs health insurance companies. Who is governing our politicians? Who is watching over them?

Health insurance companies and their Big Pharma cohorts are devilish little turds who for the privilege of being able to take risks, take advantage of us, too.

The sobering change in the government's deregulation of health insurance allowed companies to bring Americans together like rats, only to be forced or migrated from one faulty plan design to another with only selfish, profit-driven, greedy objectives in mind.

Planned obsolescence does not work in any economy. It only feeds future guarantees of failure. PPO, POS, HMO, HSA, FSA, HDHPs, and thousands of plan variations within each of these plan design alternatives are available. Are this many alternatives all that helpful to the problems that plague our healthcare system?

Is there hope or not? Try a Health Savings Account and learn how to purchase medical services with the help of transparency. It is supposed to turn doctors against each other in a price war competing for offering medical services. This is a great strategy in the new age of provider and caretaker shortages when demand for medical services is running at an all-time high. After you fund your Health Savings Account, you will be able to spend the money more wisely.

The reason we access the medical system is to get well. They say that basically no one understands their health plan completely—especially the agent who sold you it. It's nice to find out when you are really sick that you are not covered for what you actually need. Gee, isn't that sweet. When you need the health insurance protection that you are paying for, your insurance company decides what will be paid for, how, when, and to whom. Are you afraid of a single-payer Medicare-for-All system?

A light went off in some genius's head that said early detection and preventive medicine might be a good idea—*if* we don't have to pay for it. It's a relatively good idea after the insurance companies and their associated lobbying efforts complicate matters with yet another health plan type designed to keep Americans from actually getting the medical services that we really need.

Consumer-driven healthcare in its current form has no future. Last time I checked, most consumers were not doctors.

The only worthwhile model for the future of healthcare delivery in the United States is single-payer.

Removing administrative profits can keep the current system afloat while we make a benevolent transition to single-payer.

Before we get there, the underlying issues within the medical delivery system need to be corrected. Adopting evidence-based best practice preventive medical guidelines will take many years to achieve.

Isn't it better to improve our costly medical system now?

There is a significant opportunity for the United States medical delivery system to improve the quality of care through standardized oversight.

According to a survey of preventable deaths in nineteen industrialized countries, the United States scored the lowest. The countries, in order of best to worst, were France, Japan, Australia, Austria, Canada, Denmark, Finland, Germany, Greece, Ireland, Italy, Netherlands, New Zealand, Norway, Portugal, Spain, Sweden, the United Kingdom, and the United States.

No offense to any of the first eighteen countries who are our allies, friends, and global economic partners of the United States, but the United States has the most sophisticated and envied economy in the world. You might ask yourself, "How could this be happening to us? Why are we in such bad shape now?"

The kicker is that we spend considerably more money on death care than everyone of these other countries do.

One of our core problems is that we crave care in very old age when conventional wisdom screams, "Stop it! You are torturing me." Relatives can't deal with the emotions and the sick are not in the right frame of mind to make their own medical decisions. Are they? This is one of the most troubling challenges to our medical system.

Death or near death is when our medical system just pours it on in time to help us at around eighty or ninety years old so we can live three more months in a wheelchair with a feeding tube and a colostomy bag. What an awesome quality of life, don't you think? Now that is preventive care in our healthcare system today. Most of us will welcome the help to squeeze out any more time alive. Some of us would prefer not to be guinea pigs.

However, it does beat the alternative and sometimes it works. It can result in a selfish, self-serving form of torture to the patient. An older, suffering patient, who could eventually be any one of us, might think, *Thank you, America, for spending all of that money on my hopeless demise. What a big wallet—I mean heart—you have. Thanks to the medical system and some ancient values or assumptions that have no place in today's new world for allowing doctors to practice medicine on me at any cost in the last few days of life so that they practice with no regard for the quality of my life.*

Americans crave life and existence. We are strong-willed, free, generous, peaceful people. On the other hand, we love immediate gratification at almost any cost, which has already proven to be a recipe for disaster. So the $64 trillion question is what are we going to do to overhaul the U. S. medical system? Why don't you ask your doctor or insurance company for the answer?

Solutions come to us in the form of sacrifice with a purpose.

Every one of us—including Corporate America, individuals, the rich and elite, the medical system, suppliers and providers, and even the sick—need to pitch in. This is not about money. It is about your life and your health.

America must develop a medical system with a future to serve the needs of the people of this country. Americans first.

There are numerous ways to pay for any potential financial excesses that may occur. The answer is in the planning.

Where is care going and why? What about providers and caretaker shortages?

Nobody cares about my healthcare, but somebody should. Who? Me? Yes, you!

2012 U. S. Medical Plan

✓ *A preventive lifeline of care from the cradle to the grave.*

✓ *Genetic profiling* to make you a more responsible parent. A simple spit test given to every newborn to determine their genetic profile will train parents to help their children adopt a healthier existence. What a difference this will make.

✓ *Lifestyle changes* through socially conscious change. From diet to exercise, we can all do better. Stress is our silent killer.

✓ *Chronic disease control* by ending discrimination and openly accessing new tools to help resolve chronic health issues.

✓ *Low administrative costs* through single-payer as proven by CMS in Washington.

✓ *Electronic medical records* create efficiencies that go unrealized today.

✓ *Telemedicine* can lower the costs of some acute and not severe emergency-related sickness.

✓ High-tech outpatient care

✓ Pharmaceutical innovation

✓ *Transparency* leads to trust which is all but lost.

✓ *Euthanasia* can end suffering for the terminally ill.

✓ *Single-payer universal care* will insure all American citizens at lower costs with more accessible care for those citizens in need. A new U. S. identification card for all citizens who care to access healthcare. Good-bye to illegal immigrants who are stealing both opportunity and healthcare from American citizens.

✓ These are a start in the right direction.

Rising medical loss ratios at insurance companies don't tell the entire story of the worsening health insurance crisis. Insurance companies are tied to this crumbling economy. There is a cause for concern because the supposed experts at risk cannot get it under control. The underwriting curve of health insurance risk is turning the corner and going south. That means huge insurance premium increases are in store for the near future.

Rising medical loss ratios, which are simply the premium minus the actual payment of claims and general and administrative costs, are rising and will put a lot of pressure on CEOs of major health insurance companies. However, they won't be able to stop it and their profits will start to evaporate.

When health insurance executives make more than $100 million a year, we have more than forty-five million Americans without insurance and murderers in prison get free healthcare and room and board, our priorities are perverse and the trend must be reversed. Our national security depends on it.

The government must standardize all health insurance coverage similar to that of Medicare-for-All and make supplemental gap plan coverage available for those who desire more coverage than the base plan.

That would be a substantial change that scares powerful people.

We could eliminate old legislation like ERISA, federalize appropriate state mandates and remove the rest, abolish McCarron-Ferguson, and create a federal alternative health plan that opens the door to competition in the field of supplemental benefits.

My opinion is that no public or private company can compete with the federal government. Just look at the postal service. The government is the ultimate monopoly that emphasizes size matters and we can do it better and cheaper. The government—through the permission of voting Americans—also has the regulatory power and budget to enforce the New Deal for U. S. Healthcare. Reward America and its wonderful citizens with the New Deal for U. S. Healthcare and support our regrouping as a country to compete in the global world. Healthcare is a right. We need it that way.

Recognize quality and create incentives for healthy living. Reward providers who—given all of the risk factors—elevate the quality of a patient's health throughout their lifetime. Penalize all vendors for nonperformance. Punish fraud. A single-payer healthcare system will not only save 30 percent of every healthcare dollar, it could put the lid on the costs associated with uncoordinated care in chronic disease management.

Did you know that most Americans with diabetes have no idea of the most up-to-date treatment options?

We are given hope by the medical system only when we are sick.

What about proactive preparation for the diseases we may be genetically predisposed to from birth?

Because healthcare is big business, it is not about health at all, it is about profiting from risk.

Education is the only way to promote and force change. It is too bad that Washington rhetoric wastes so much money.

Just do it.

What happened to accountability? The core of America's existence in the world depends on fixing this aspect of our economy and our lives. America needs this change to move forward. Sure, there will be disappointments and disillusion along the way. That is the nature of change. With change comes uncertainty. However, we are not guessing—we are resolving.

It's the end of the world for the current U. S. healthcare system.

Change is going to come. It is taking place before your very eyes. America is changing for the better.

We are spreading our generosity to our own citizens through the most essential social program.

Healthcare where we are all protected is supportive of market and economic dynamics for our competitive future.

Although there are many battles ahead, they will be swept under by the forces of dynamic and innovative change. Order will be restored by the New Deal for U. S. Healthcare within the next twenty years. America's world dominance in certain areas will reemerge as we gear up for the most important change in our economic history.

We are approaching crisis mode where America performs best. United as we stand, let's get this done so our children and their children can benefit from the advantages that America has to offer its people.

What kind of healthcare system will we have in twenty years that is so much better than today? A healthcare system that embraces coordinated care incorporating all medical advances to keep Americans well.

Euthanasia and End-of-Life Care

Why does common sense always seem to lose this battle? Either way, the victim is truly the patient. Death is always hard to accept for loved ones. Our healthcare system has trained Americans to believe that life at any cost—regardless of the quality of life—is well worth it. When a doctor or institution gives relatives and friends of terminally ill patients hope, it is a crime. It is a difficult line to draw for which no one wants to take responsibility. Kevorkian believed in mature decision making on behalf of the terminally ill. Many questioned his motives as though he were a criminal psychopathic physician killing people. Dr. Kevorkian might have been the most compassionate doctor in the last fifty years.

Although many people admire the strength exhibited by terminally ill patients, where do we, their appointed decision makers, draw the line? Did you know that 27 percent of Medicare budget is spent on end-of-life care?

Do we honor a terminally ill patient's do-not-resuscitate orders?

What if they don't have a will?

Are they conscious?

Are they comatose?

Are they cash payers beyond what their insurance coverage provides in the way of protection?

Do they have insurance protection at all?

What are the patient's chances for survival?

How old is this patient?

Do we know if they are suffering?

What kind of life quality will they have should they miraculously survive?

How long or at what point should respiration or other life support systems be removed?

What do we do then?

How long is an appropriate hospitalization for the terminally ill?

Why can't Americans grow up and draw some lines?

Why did we let religion influence healthcare?

Immaturity about death is a terrible weakness. Living life to its fullest is a great strength. Life does not last forever. It is up to you to live it.

To examine end-of-life care purely from a financial standpoint is sickening. What an atrocious rip off. Americans pay seriously for end-of-life surgical procedures and hospitalization. Is that honoring the people we love?

Accountability in medicine is not as it is for most of us that are working people. Most of the money for seniors and the uninsured comes from American taxpayers who have no idea how the money they pay the government is being spent.

Medicare and Medicaid are excellent programs that have a significant impact on American lives. These programs can be improved to take into account the advances in medical science and the growth of our population. These entitlement programs recognized the needs of elderly Americans, those with medical disabilities, and Americans who have fallen on hard economic times.

It is too bad that these public programs were never meant to cover the entire population. However, one can see from the way our medical system works that limits on care associated with these programs are loosely held together. The reimbursement game for providing medical services has been mastered by the provider side of the medical industry.

The provider side of the healthcare business has focused so much on productivity that they lost the unique feel for human life that once demonstrated kindness, empathy, and quality-of-life standards.

Practicing medicine at any cost in America must stop.

One more year or month of life could cost a million dollars. Is it fair to spread that among all taxpayers? What if that was you? We have some difficult decisions to make in light of medical science and discovery. Eternal life does not exist for humans. Life is short and Americans enjoy their freedom.

Euthanasia solves problems associated with terminally ill patients.

It is not innovative, but very realistic.

There are numerous studies that paint a very inaccurate picture of what is going on in healthcare, health insurance, and the U. S. healthcare system.

The current system cannot sustain itself.

Where are the newspapers and politicians digging up these manipulative statistics?

Everything is not okay. We all understand that. Most polls show that Americans believe the healthcare system must change.

Sure, we have 45 million uninsured Americans, but they are only a small part of the problem. Knowledge is power. Learn and become powerful. Don't let insurance companies, the medical system, and pharmaceutical companies, the U. S. government and even your employer lie to you.

The truth is that healthcare advances are light years ahead of where they were just twenty years ago. The healthcare system in America has many good points. The care is excellent in some places in our disjointed system. Otherwise it can really suck. For instance, when you are stuck or live in a rural part of America, it is likely that the centers of medical excellence are far away. Most Americans get their healthcare delivered locally or regionally. What about you? If you needed serious care and had a small window of time, what would you do? In an emergency or for different degrees of medical need, where would you go and what doctor would you use?

You can find out what treatment alternatives are available and who the most appropriate facilities and doctors are to treat your condition. It takes time and commitment. It is especially difficult when you are sick.

How do you help yourself when you are a victim of the healthcare system or in trouble with your health or financially?

Most of my clients call me, and I take care of it. I am an expert at chasing down health insurance reimbursement for my clients who have become victims of their insurance company and are technically covered.

There are so many ways to help oneself within our current healthcare system. First, understand that healthcare disasters can happen to a fetus, an infant, a child, an adult, or the elderly. Welcome to reality.

Now, what can you do about it?

How healthy are you now?

What is your family history of disease?

Do you want to stay healthy or end up in a hospital and then a nursing home?

Have you ever been in a nursing home?

What kind of prevention are you practicing?

Who is in your healthcare network for an unexpected crisis?

Where do you go in the event of a serious emergency?

What about a nonlife-threatening emergency?

When is the last time you had a physical?

Do you know what your parents and grandparents health history was and why?

The Genetic Information Act should protect you from discrimination. We are progressing at a snail's pace.

What should you do with the information that you collect to answer these questions? Update it every year.

Americans would be a lot more focused on their health if their care was provided in an organized, simple, more effective delivery system that stressed prevention through early detection and lifestyle changes.

Administering one plan through a single-payer approach would enable healthcare providers to focus on quality care issues instead of reimbursement and other red tape. Providers could exceed expectations without the worry of being sued.

We could offer all Americans a choice of the current Federal Employee Health Benefits Plans.

What about one comprehensive Medicare-like benefit for all?

That would at least placate the insurance lobbies and their adversaries … temporarily.

A few choice carriers could compete for the business. Congress could stop wasting time on the uninsured and get back to creating pathways to innovation within a medical program that creates gap coverage for those who can afford greater protection. We do have to absorb the uninsured. The challenge is how. We have to fix the medical side of the system alongside the lower administrative costs through technology gains that we will eventually realize.

Access to care will get better. Your perception is your reality. Access to necessary medical care should be the same as private programs and social programs that exist today within the current system. Don't give up on change. Many positive aspects of the medical delivery system won't change except that hospitals, suppliers, and other providers will not be able to bill taxpaying citizens non-negotiated, unjustifiable rip-off rates. They need to be held accountable for delivering the best possible practiced care. Eventually, the entire medical system can be everything it is capable of being without destroying what is good about it. It is all about accountability.

America is not Canada or England or even France.

Those countries have their own medical systems. Some aspects of their systems are good and some are bad. France has a nice working medical system that most of its citizens are very happy with. America is larger, is much more resilient, and has a stronger economy—even in our worst recession—than other countries that have socialized medical programs.

The number of places Americans can access care is quite remarkable. I do not believe it was only profit that drove access. Demand for medical services and the overabundance of access to medical delivery in our country is something that is unique, expensive, and wasteful in our capitalistic democracy. The perception that more is better in medicine could have worked if it simply implied wellness keeps you healthy. We still have to tame the healthcare utilization curve through efficiencies, medical innovation, chronic disease education, and early intervention through genetic studies.

What does the future hold for Americans and healthcare?

Health information technology

Transparency

Medical advances

Alternative Medicine

Cost controls

A different kind of medical access

Physician shortages

Hospital bankruptcies

Single-payer healthcare

Nursing shortages

CNA and home health aide shortages

Advanced genetic testing objectives

Privatized or socialized … it's all about to change

Who are the real winners and losers?

Where do we go from here?

Will it be enough?

Don't our politicians owe us an explanation about how they intend to solve our problems instead of the rhetoric of telling us what our problems are as a nation? We know that the open checkbook is going to get us in trouble. We already know and are feeling it financially and emotionally.

If you were forced to run the government, would you allow the money to be spent frivolously, permit rampant corruption, and forget about the majority of the people you are supposed to represent? Where is all of the money being spent? Insurance is supposed to be about protection. So is the government—in addition to many other services.

Here is a worthy strategy for change:

Identify the enemy. We did that. Your employer is not the enemy, though they can sometimes appear that way. Believe it or not, they are part of the problem and the implications of change scare large employers. Your employer is an advocate of promoting better healthcare for employees when they offer a group plan. Why? Because, employers contribute financially to your health plan, don't they? It is not an employee right to have health insurance unless you are eligible for a plan that your employer offers. When offered employer-sponsored group health insurance from an employer, most Americans choose that option. There are also many Americans who purchase individual health insurance privately and on their own. Individual coverage can be less expensive in many cases because it is subject to medical underwriting. Many Americans struggle with their contributions to pay the healthcare premium to begin with—even before doctor, hospital, and prescription co-pays, deductibles, and other out-of-pocket expenses. Unless your earnings are at or below the criteria for public assistance, you will have to pay toward or pay all of your health insurance premiums.

Depending on the state that you reside in and your income level, your children might be able to access public programs—even if you have coverage offered through your employer. Isn't that crazy? Your rights as an American are different depending on the state you live in.

How united is that? Aren't we the United States? On March 9, 1945, the McCarran-Ferguson Act was passed by Congress. It allows state law to regulate the business of insurance without federal government interference. Among others, it allows for

➤ the state regulation of insurance,

➤ states to establish mandatory licensing requirements, and

➤ preservation of certain state laws of insurance.

Senator McCain seemed to be proposing Americans should pay for their own healthcare coverage and perhaps abandon their corporate coverage. Your reward would be a personal tax deduction. What a disaster! Although the idea of repealing the McCarran-Ferguson act for selling coverage interstate would be a good idea, McCain's overall proposal will only exacerbate the uninsured and insured problem. Allowing insurance to be federally regulated and sold interstate is the excellent part of his proposal. Many of us have concrete solutions to contribute.

The 2008 presidential elections led to no solutions. None of the candidates has ever paved the way to Americans understanding how the healthcare system will get better and less expensive. No details mean no plans.

Now, with that being said, when you get sick, Americans are sure as hell glad that there are some great doctors—most of the time—to help us get well. Unfortunately, a small sampling often taints the reputation of an entire field. Doctors do not enjoy the godlike status they had in previous generations. It does take a high level of intelligence, an excellent attitude, years of experience practicing medicine, and a commitment to continued study and research to be a great diagnostician.

Most Americans would prefer to have health insurance protection or some form of protection from catastrophic financial loss due to being sick. The problem is that Americans don't want to pay for it—at least directly. However, we won't object to paying for an efficient healthcare system through taxes—provided the right incentives to the Medical industry lead to more favorable outcomes at a better price.

Get rid of health insurance companies altogether. They can compete in related markets and supplements.

The majority of Americans like our healthcare delivery system, but don't like their insurance company. Many do not trust the government.

If we don't trust the government, why did we elect them in the first place? Do you trust your health insurance company more?

For those of you that have been sick, you are sure glad the insurance company was there to protect you. An insurance company decides your fate as opposed to the government. Medicare is the most generous of all insurance plans. Its only shortfall came about as a result of medical and pharmaceutical advances that could not have been imagined in 1965.

What difference does it make? Would you prefer your healthcare be governed by your health insurance company monopoly or through the government?

By the way, only a few other countries in the world could afford America's medical delivery system. Even those few that could, don't want it. Why? The answer is simple. Our healthcare system is too expensive and designed to fail. It is built on ancient principles that include planned obsolescence. You can't endorse new technologies without building an infrastructure to support them. Our fragmented medical and insurance systems are adversarial and unproductive. Americans continue to pay the price for inefficient medicine financially as illustrated by our third world like survival statistics.

We are all going to die some day. Develop a system that strongly encourages longevity through healthy living as opposed to the current crisis-oriented approach that preys on our inevitable demise. America is approaching the biggest shortage of doctors and nurses versus our needs in our history. In every weakness is an opportunity to advance or exploit. We need to build a new system that embraces medical advances, education, and technology. The upcoming provider shortage couldn't come at a worse time. Evidence-based medicine, transparency, and electronic medical records are only part of the new solution. They are the most obvious, but not the most creative. We need to move swiftly toward the new healthcare system. There are so many ways to fund healthcare for all Americans that it is not funny. In fact, we already do. Everyone has something to say about where the funding has to come from. Let's bite the bullet and stop kidding ourselves. There are numerous ways to raise additional funds to bring about swift change.

Americans are energy-consuming pigs. How do you kill two birds with one stone here? Gasoline is so expensive, but a fifty-cent-per-gallon tax, to be used for healthcare and alternative fuel research at the pump would do it. A corporate luxury tax on all oil companies would help. Those record-breaking profits in an industry that feeds terrorism and weakens America should be used for advancing what is good for our country and people. Do you have any idea how your tax money is spent? The people you elect know. Americans should curtail the use of oil, which only contributes financially to rogue governments who sponsor terrorism and want to hurt America. Eat green and healthy, use alternative fuels, get exercise, and stay away from smoking, fast food, soda, and other destructive foods. This is a process where America can self-actualize and get back to showing the rest of the world why we are who we are.

Personal change is simply fundamental to correcting the behavior of large monopolistic entities that control abusive industries and our lives. What can you do?

Do you believe that you are powerful enough to change your own behavior? Unfortunately, most of us do not. Can you learn how? Yes.

Become aware and educated on what healthcare means to you. Seek assistance.

1) Prepare for the war on medical terrorism.

2) Declare war. Put a plan into action. We can no longer settle for diplomacy. Be on the side of human rights.

3) Seek out, defeat, and destroy all of the wasteful ancient principles of how medical care is provided and administered. They have no place in an advanced society. Get in shape and get healthy.

4) Restore order. There is so much to do and so many parts are moving in the wrong direction.

Where do we start?

Well, that depends on your age and your health. However, we will settle for a general approach that everyone can build on to identify his or her enemies within our healthcare system and get on the right track.

The enemy has disguised itself in so many different ways. The resilient chameleonlike enemy has no conscience. The enemy does not like change.

You are confused about your insurance and the healthcare system by design. Whatever forms the enemy takes, as a consumer and utilizer of the U. S. medical system, you must understand how it works and where you can make a difference. This new knowledge might someday save your life or prevent financial catastrophe.

Remember that your health is a gift. Protect it!

Are you your own worst enemy? Are you resistant to change? Change is not easy to accomplish—whether it is systematic or personal. What you ask of our healthcare system, you must demand of yourself, too. Control starts with your own life. What can you do differently in order to defeat the enemy?

Educate yourself. Didn't your momma tell you that? Are you satisfied with your understanding of the health plan benefits that you have? Do you have health insurance? Which type of coverage? Individual or group coverage? What type of plan design? Do you understand how your plan really works? Does your agent? I doubt it.

What is the purpose of having health insurance?

Some would argue that it is only for catastrophic financial protection. I beg to differ. The opportunities that premiums afford us go deeper than financial protection. We have an expectation level of not only protection, but also performance.

Who is supposed to perform? The insurance company, the doctor, hospital, lab, billing company, collection agency, the government, or you?

Insurance companies take risks and tell us that they expect to make a modest profit—after paying enormous salaries and bonuses to top brass and their respective lobbying firms. However, many insurance companies are poorly run and have overwhelmingly high overhead. Corporate greed has driven the general and administrative expenses of insurance companies to deplorable levels. How much of every healthcare dollar is spent to run these companies? CEOs are taking home outrageous amounts of pay, stock incentives, and other forms of compensation and shareholders and boards of directors are letting them get away with it. Meanwhile, money to pay for better care is not there. Just look at this horrible example of corporate greed with the nation's largest managed care conglomerate.

I wrote this blog on Thursday, March 8, 2007.

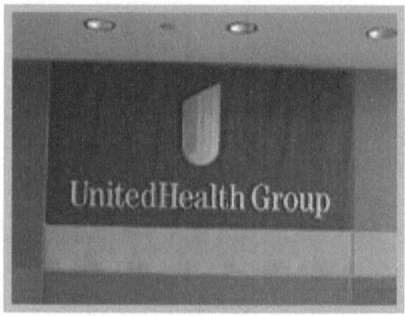

Where does the U. S. government draw the line on corporate greed?

Where does the U. S. government draw the line on corporate greed when it comes to America's most talked about social problem: health insurance?

United Health Group, the largest U. S. health insurance company continues to reward shareholders at the expense of its commercial and Medicare customers. This earnings report demonstrates the U. S. government's level of tolerance for letting corporate giants in health insurance get away with unethical standards that seem to apply only to them. A 35 percent profit margin in health insurance is obscene by most standards. No wonder there are so many without health insurance. Where is that money going? It is certainly not going in to medical care for members of their health plans. Many of UHC's members are burdened by the accelerated cost-shifting in the consumer-driven plans that they are market leaders in, while UHC continues to reap huge profits. This is doing nothing to resolve problems within the U. S. healthcare system. Consumer-driven plans have impacted utilization patterns of members. Instead of doing the right thing, as the largest player in the field, UHC's greed to squeeze profits is placing an enormous financial burden on members of their plans. Consumer-driven plans have impacted utilization patterns of members. Perhaps members are not accessing unnecessary medical care. However, what if members are avoiding care because of high deductibles? We already know that avoiding care leads to more significant costs later on. Is this really helping anyone? Do consumer-driven plans do anything more than increase insurance company profits? In the long run, maybe yes.

Health insurance companies want to change their insureds' behavior toward accessing medical care. Why aren't health insurance companies lowering premiums significantly for those that are more risk-tolerant by electing consumer-driven plans, when there is so much profit to be made? Is it greed? If UHC and its competitors are trying to change the medical utilization patterns of members, where is the reward for the premium-paying members?

So insurance companies create plan designs that change consumer behavior due to cost-shifting, which means that we as consumers pay a larger portion of the healthcare expenses because all insurance company plan designs incorporate cost-shifting in to their very nature. The reason we have so much over utilization of medical services in this country is largely by design. From managed care to consumerism, how do you like forced migration? Ever feel like a rat in a maze? Now the insurance companies with the help of Uncle Sam are trying to force

Americans into Health Savings Accounts. Be wary of them. HSAs are poison unless you are rich and/or healthy. They may save money in the short run, but the long-term strategy is flawed. Providers don't like them either because the high deductibles are making medical debt more difficult to collect. Most Americans simply cannot afford high-deductible health insurance. Low co-pays and low out-of-pocket costs associated with HMOs were the model that the insurance companies and employers wanted. Supply-and-demand theory in medicine puts a price on human life. Hey, all you right-to-lifers, is it worth it? Is health insurance coverage a right or a privilege? Are you worth it? Is it all worth it? Who determines that? You, a loved one, an insurance company, the medical caregiver, or the U. S. government? Mandatory health insurance coverage? We will see about that. America cannot afford to overpay while we overutilize the medical system. Cost is going to have to be addressed as soon as possible. Mandatory, universal or whatever label is in vogue at the particular moment you are reading this takes universal changes. That means many huge changes that will affect the future of America for a long time. If there is no government takeover of healthcare or health insurance, how are Americans going to be able to afford the current trend in twenty years? What will our economy look like in twenty years? Our health is our wealth. Our competitiveness can only be as good as our preparedness. We are no longer dominant in everything. America has to compete against the up-and-comers who have everything to gain and nothing to lose. The next twenty years are the world series of economic dominance. American healthcare must be secure—just like our borders. A new system of healthcare would do just that. One plan for all, where eligibility is determined through U. S. citizenship. What is wrong with that? Oh, it is too easy. Single-payer resolves immigration issues at the same time. Oh, that is too efficient.

What about association health plans for small businesses or individuals? They exist for the privileged few. AARP is an association. The current underlying health insurer for AARP is United Healthcare. Aetna is now their early retiree solution from ages 50–64. Every Professional Employer Organization (PEO) is an association helping businesses run effectively. What about no underwriting or preexisting conditions? Nobody is listening to the American public. We need financial relief. Our savings rate is at an all-time low, and our expenses are running higher than ever. America is on the verge of financial catastrophe. Either way, I am betting on America. Americans will respond to their future needs when forced to.

Watch out for the free market correction coming in healthcare.

There is nothing but more problems coming until we fix what we can now and plan for the future. We need to regroup and stay united to believe that Americans control their healthcare future. Just look at some statistics from the 2007 study from the Employee Benefit Research Institute.

Healthcare is not a funny topic—although it can be when we are speaking about nonlife-threatening issues. Still healthcare can be dry and serious. Staying fit and being conscious of eating and nutrition can only benefit your health. There are many Web sites with scary statistics. Take an interest and I am sure you will find statistics that will frighten you. Healthcare needs to be restructured to meet the needs of our future generations. We are behind the curve here.

Stakeholders have so much representation in all the right places that we face gridlock. The only system that can work for America is a single-payer system. Americans want our cake and we want to eat it. Our unrealistic expectations will never bring about complete satisfaction. The senseless rhetoric against single-payer comes from stakeholders and the wealthy who could buy gap plans to increase their own particular coverage anyway. What has to happen will consist of numerous changes that will take place over the next ten to twenty years.

However, changes start with you.

Those of you who are interested and motivated enough will think of some way that you can make a difference—even a very small difference. Perhaps, a healthy diet or more exercise. Making sure your children are doing the right thing. Maybe those of you that are bold enough and actually think your vote could make a difference by exercising it wisely (no pun intended!). I couldn't be more serious.

What is stopping you from taking a walk, controlling portions instead of overeating, or reading about care alternatives? These all could accelerate your healing process and make you feel better. Could you possibly be so naïve as to think that the providers who treat and advise you have a monopoly on all prognoses?

Try these Web sites that I like:

www. mayoclinic. com

www. clevelandclinic. com

www. nih. com

www. ebri. com

The list can be expanded so easily. Just Google it, put in your question, disease or condition, exercise physiology, mental health, etc. So much information that we take for granted is right at our fingertips.

I already told you that if a provider is not online with all of the companies they get reimbursed from, they should not be allowed to practice medicine. Are we in the Stone Age? With that should come electronic medical records and evidence-based medicine practice guidelines. You don't want to get well, do you? Then do something about it.

Doctors and insurance companies attempt to control our freedom. Doctors want to be paid up front, and insurance companies make us conform to meet their standards of access. Access to doctors and hospitals is generally easy as long as you follow the rules and live in a region where healthcare is accessible. Rural areas are not on equal ground with city dwellers. Unfortunately this phenomenon mostly affects those with lower incomes and minorities. It also affects all of us when we are somewhere that does not meet our medical needs at the time.

The out-of-pocket costs for a medical encounter could be extremely costly if you do not access the insurance company's network. The health insurance industry is now trying to correct its miscalculations and manipulate the way Americans access system, so they can make more money and keep premiums reasonable. The consumer-driven movement is not about consumers; it's about insurance companies driving the way Americans interact with the medical system. We are just the victims. Thanks a lot.

Health insurance companies are the enemy.

They have free reign to play with our lives. Health insurance companies feel that by taking risk, they own us. If we break the rules, they do not pay. If you incur a substantial claim, it has to be submitted properly by the doctor, hospital, or lab—and you better follow up with the insurance company when you start getting bills and collection letters like crazy. Don't expect the medical billing or claims to be filed properly.

Don't pay any bills until you call the customer service line at the health insurance company and go over every bill and explanation of benefits in detail. They can be very helpful. Write down the time and person's name with whom you spoke. Just try to have some patience. If you don't get any cooperation, you may have a problem. Try your employee benefits or human resource department. If they are not available to you, ask to speak with your insurance agent, broker, or consultant. If they have the skills and knowledge, they should be willing to negotiate on your behalf. If not, maybe you should talk to someone in your company who cares. After reading this book, you will be able to speak up for yourself, intelligently about our healthcare system and how you are treated should you need medical services.

I would like anyone with a story they would like to tell about the healthcare system to send it to my e-mail address at lsx100@yahoo.com. I would like to help any company that is not getting the best representation. Thank you.

What about other potential enemies? You have to watch your back and cover your ass. Have you ever heard that? It is especially true when it comes to health insurance.

The government is a stumbling block—even though Uncle Sam usually tries to protect us. Their intentions are sometimes good, but the road to hell is paved with good intentions. They need to get their act together.

What role does the government play in our healthcare system and how does that effect me?

The role of the federal and state governments is critical when it comes to health insurance. The Center for Medicare and Medicaid Services really are not bad social programs. Communication and education of changes to these programs and how they impact the majority of Americans who belong to these programs is very effective. Just look at how many Americans qualify for these public or socialized programs and don't know they qualify. What about the Medicare Part D debacle? The drug benefits were first dollar with a deductible coming after you exhausted the first dollar allowance. Then, after satisfying that deductible, you were covered like you were at the beginning—prior to incurring the deductible. Benefit, deductible, benefit. Not as complicated as everyone made it. Was it even necessary to be that complicated? The problem always gets down to cost.

Drugs cost too much in this country. That must change immediately because our current system has grown dependent on Big Pharma in an unconstructive kind of way. They are simply ripping off American taxpayers and should be regulated. Why is it that other countries in which U. S. pharmaceutical companies compete are being supplemented in cost by American taxpayers. That is abuse and should not be tolerated by our government. Shorten patent protection.

The McCarran-Ferguson Act was a mistake and single-handedly changed the vision of a single-payer system for decades to come. Regionalization of healthcare and access are always going to pose a challenge in rural areas. Getting around the United States is not very difficult. Only when a severe emergency occurs in a rural area is access a problem. Otherwise, higher quality institutions tend to be located in major cities and very populated areas. Access to them may be limited but they are there. Is that so different from the care offered in other countries? That could change for the better with a new U. S. single-payer medical program. We shall see what stumbling blocks are encountered as Congress moves toward change in America's healthcare system.

The focus of the 2008 political candidates on the uninsured shows us how out of touch they are with the majority of Americans who are insured and are still getting shafted by a wasteful and error-laden system—not to mention the obscene administrative costs in the private sector.

Are we really that naïve that we will allow this to continue?

The U. S. healthcare system will be a single-payer system. It is only a matter of time.

There will be a shakeout among providers much the way it happened with pharmacies. Big Pharma will be encouraged to make bacteria-fighting drugs regardless of profit because the government will sponsor it. We have no choice. Blood replacements are a priority too. I can't list all of the areas that need improvement because that is a book in itself.

The quality of healthcare has nothing to do with a single-payer. In fact, I believe that the quality of medical delivery will improve greatly under single-payer. The reason for single-payer is that standardization provides a much-needed structure for easier, less expensive and more effective oversight. Administrative costs savings will be considerable. Quality studies that are evidence-based with scientific support have a future in our healthcare system. All providers need to be online with payers so the patient does not have to endure endless red tape. Otherwise they should not be practicing medicine. Yes—not practicing on you. They deserved to get paid when services are delivered.

Let's give doctors a little reprieve. Doctors go through at least six years of college and grad school. They only collect 70 percent of their receivables on average nationally (that would be like you working forty-five hours and getting paid for thirty-two) and pay outrageous amounts of money for malpractice insurance while paying back their student loans. Through hard work, physicians eventually get ahead of the curve. Suppliers and other beneficiaries of treating the sick do quite well financially along with physicians or providers when they are fairly reimbursed. However, we still need them—and apparently quite badly. Demand is out of control and largely by design. It is no coincidence that demand for medical services is out of control and supply is somewhat limited. Many things contributed to our insatiable appetite for healthcare.

What can America do about cost and demand? We could deprive the sick of medical care or we could not pay medical bills. What are the other options?

Entitlement programs can really upset Americans who work their butts off, pay taxes, and contribute their time to better our country. Most Americans support the premise that our healthcare system needs change. There is still hope for private industry in the medical field, but do you want profit objectives to influence the healthcare that you receive—or do you simply want to access the best possible healthcare for whatever ails you at that time and place within reason?

Is the government going to make things worse than they already are for us in healthcare? Most Americans have a fairly high degree of satisfaction with our healthcare system. It is just too expensive. Whether you work for a Fortune 1000 company or the government, you probably have health insurance coverage. If you work for a small company, the odds of having a health plan offered to you are dramatically lower. Contributions to premiums in small group health plans usually require a higher contribution from the employee with little choice of plan design. The cost of employer-sponsored health insurance coverage has been out of hand for a decade. The cherry picking individual plan model goes against everything that must be included for costs to be fair and under control.

Spreading risk across the entire population, having a base plan of coverage similar to a Medicare plan for all of those who qualify, limiting certain benefits, creating incentives for healthy living, revamping the medical reimbursement code to all providers, suppliers, and pharmaceutical manufacturers, and changing to a single-payer approach will save trillions of dollars over the next two decades and greatly improve morbidity and mortality rates.

It will take everything we have as a nation to make this happen. America must heal its broken healthcare system. There are many issues that affect the way the system works. They involve laws and statutes and lots of money, jobs, ethics, and morals. This model of healthcare that I am proposing is not about losing jobs or just another entitlement program. It is about improving the lives of all Americans. It has nothing to do with democracy or capitalism. It has everything to do with doing the right thing for our children's future.

American politics are getting in the way of progress.

Capitalism will benefit greatly. One huge door must close and another will open through innovation and achievement. Isn't that what the free market is about?

Americans deserve their healthcare to be a right.

Would it be so bad if we amended the Constitution? Americans are the world's most productive people. We need a break from ourselves. Taxes will pay for the new system. There is no lying about that. We already pay for it, so the money is there and can be used more effectively.

Stop worrying about other country's socialized healthcare systems and concentrate on how our system works, how it can improve, and what we need to do in what time line to get there.

What we can do to honor and retain the best aspects of our broken fragmented privatized system of care while we move toward a more effective and efficient system where all of us are covered? Lack of coordination in our fragmented system leads to medical errors for far too many insured Americans.

Americans are seeking protection through insurance from statistical odds of financial catastrophe. With all of the cost-shifting in plan designs such as Health Savings Accounts and other plans with very high co-payments and large deductibles, Americans are bearing the brunt of the financial problems that plague the system. Basically, the health insurance industry forced changes and by assuming more risk, insurance companies took more control. They caused the breakdown in the medical system that is worsening by the day.

Americans are victims of claims denials for various reasons. All plans have limits. Medicare and gap plans have standardized limits. The only confusion in Medicare is from the HMOs. Insurance companies are always seeking ways to deny or refuse coverage for claims. That is part of their business. It ain't pretty—but it is *very* profitable. If you were to research the CEO pay at the ten largest managed care and health insurance companies, you would be incredibly disappointed at the greed level. Meanwhile the system continues to break down. Where is their commitment? What—or who—are their priorities?

If federal legislators know what to do (since most progressive states are struggling with the poor results of their efforts to reform healthcare), why the inertia? Money, debate, or lobbying dollars?

It is a challenge to pick a spot to start endorsing agreed upon changes, but we just came up with $700 billion in paper money to save our economy. My estimate is that will be the first of two more progressively larger bailouts. When America is in a crisis, it is amazing how congressmen feel compelled to pass legislation that may be bad for our country and our future.

Healthcare experts agree on most of the obvious technological advances being applied to the healthcare system or that are yet to come. The government should fix the medical delivery shortfalls in reimbursement philosophy and methodology prior to turning everything else upside down. When we insert the proper incentives on medical delivery at all levels, the way medicine is practiced will change for the better.

Doctors, hospitals, pharmacies, and any other providers of medical services should all be online 24/7 with a single-payer in order to practice medicine in this country. The changes in reimbursement will identify where immediate intervention is called for.

Insurance companies have reported for decades that 80 percent of the claims payments are generated by 20 percent of their membership. It is actually fairly close. We know that their current chronic disease management and education programs are weak and have not proved effective. There are a high number of prescriptions not being filled by chronically ill patients. Some employers are taking invasive approaches to manage their sickest employees. Although a degree of privacy is being breached by some employer-sponsored plans governed under ERISA, a federal law that supersedes most state laws pertaining to health insurance, as long as there is no discrimination evident, most sick and employed Americans should welcome the help.

America is supposed to be the world's leader in human rights.

If Americans are such advocates of human rights, why don't we recognize healthcare as an American right?

American politicians are so busy investing their time protecting our American interests in other country's affairs that they forgot about their own. Be well and enjoy what life has to offer. Stay or get healthy. Thank you for believing in your health.

Support a constitutional amendment that guarantees healthcare for all American citizens. America must initiate and pass the New Deal for U. S. Healthcare through a constitutional amendment. There is no better time than now. No political party owns healthcare reform—the citizens of America do.

The lifestyles of Americans need to transform. Freedom gives us the power to do anything. We are an information-rich society. Every Americans eventually needs to live up to our own health potential by embracing the advancement of medical information around us that educates us and promotes healthy living. Let a welcomed transformation of the American healthcare system begin. The advancing, remarkable, and ideological practice of medicine eventually run down by insurance companies to the logical, evidence-based, practical single-payer model, where every American knows how their healthcare system works. From suppliers to providers to institutions to the patient side, everyone will know one system. That is an excellent place to start the transformation. Risk is born by all citizens. There are limits on private insurance and there will be limits on single-payer insurance for all Americans. No more negotiating with your insurance company to get the coverage you are paying for and may actually need. This is about human rights. Every American wins.

What is wrong with healthcare?

Maybe we should start with what is right about healthcare in America. We have access to numerous medical advances through new procedures and drugs that are keeping many sick Americans well.

So what's wrong?

American are immature about death and don't understand their rights to medical care when they are alive and well.

Cost, quality, human rights, and profit have no correlation.

We have a supply-and-demand problem.

Congress is lost on the healthcare issue. Just look at the recent Medicare cost issue. Insurance companies create a gap and we all pay more. Insurance companies reimburse your doctor 30–50 percent less than our government pays for the same services. AARP is not the only supplemental medicare gap plan supplier. They are an association health plan. Remember, your health insurance company spent millions of dollars lobbying against association health care coverage. Then … All medicare gap plans have standardized coverage, Plan E is Plan E from any insurance companies that are approved by the Centers for Medicare and Medicaid. There may be less expensive alternatives to AARP for the same coverage! If you don't know that, then buyer beware.

Administrative costs from the health insurance or the risk industry feed the greedy and rob the needy of money originally slated for healthcare expenses of their insured populations.

Underwriting and pre-existing conditions exclusions keep Americans from getting the care they need because the profits from discriminatory and predatory cherry picking of applicants makes insurance executives richer and more powerful.

American health information technology is too slow in responding to the emerging needs of the consolidating factors affecting medical costs.

There are too many avoidable medical errors. That in itself is a type of terrorism that America imposes on itself. The statistics of medical error and death are very disturbing.

We have a procedure-driven and crisis-oriented medical system of care delivery in which providers have the nerve to complain about reimbursement. Some have a right and some do not. Everybody in medicine is chasing the almighty dollar. We are faced with a huge opportunity to change the philosophy about helping your fellow man instead of all of the aggression people have toward one another.

Americans are burdened with too many insurance plan designs to choose from for individuals and employees. In fact, employees and individuals find health insurance very confusing. That is by design. Now you won't actually know how you are covered should you need medical attention for an illness or a disease until it happens to you—and it will. I can guarantee it.

The employer-sponsored and individual models are ready for extinction. History will show how devious, insatiable CEOs sucked the blood out of the U. S. free markets. Healthcare reform will have its day.

No American should go without insurance protection. Better yet, every American should have healthcare protection as a right.

Does evidence-based medicine and health information technology seem too cumbersome, complicated, and costly for medical providers? Doctors and care providers should not be able to practice medicine in any form unless they are online with their vendors and have access to complete medical history data. Do you know why most doctors are bad diagnosticians? Maybe they are unorganized and can't spend the time necessary to make better diagnosis. They don't have all of the information to diagnose and make a prognosis at their fingertips. But, they will under single payor.

States have too much control, which accounts for all of the inconsistency in health insurance. The government needs to standardize medicine. Standardization works very well with Medicare. Even gap coverage is standardized in Medicare. I know that the Republicans have tried to derail Medicare because they have a different agenda—and only they know it. It is some imaginary thing that will make everything better. It is not regulation or enforcement? How can so many people be wrong? Wake up out there.

What is really wrong with the healthcare in the United States is that our lame-duck Congress will never pass useful legislation in time to take effect before the crisis spirals out of control. That has become the American way. They will probably rush some healthcare legislation thru now that they have control of Congress. Please be careful and use restraint.

The levees are breaking, and Congress will wait until half of America is drowning financially before they intervene in some halfhearted, useless way.

There is a consequence for every action or inaction. I hope we can swim our way out of this evil financial tsunami. Somebody has to pay the price.

Good-bye to America as we knew it. We are going to build a bigger and better model for the future.

Access to healthcare in American will eventually become a constitutional right. Your life should be blessed with excellent health and happiness. Then, when your time has come, as it does for every living thing, I hope they let you die peacefully. Amen.

Euthanasia is scary if you are not the one making the decision. We all want to live forever—unless we are depressed, in pain, incapacitated, or grieving. Suicide is a dark and dirty subject. Let's separate that completely. Suicide is an abomination and terrible. Euthanasia is the freedom to choose. It should be part of a living will. Terminal loss of quality of life should grant you the right of no return—especially at the cost of some self-fulfilling medical profit … not prophet or sage like. Where is the dignity in helplessness? The money is in death and prevention of it at the very end of your life. Those that practice it are not feeling the effects of this financial devastation. Where do they get the nerve?

That is the incentive. It's too little, too late.

Would you rather live a healthier life or a sicker and longer life? Be proactive about your lifestyle and stay well. This is it.

www.ingramcontent.com/pod-product-compliance
Lightning Source LLC
Chambersburg PA
CBHW032019170526
45157CB00002B/776